...ddresses an underserved area, sexual ...alth, in patients undergoing ...eatment for prostate cancer. The ...rspective and information content ...ovides a tremendous resource for men ...nd their partners confronting this ...mmon disease.

—Dr. Arthur L. Burnett,
Director, Male Sexual
HealthClinic, The
Johns Hopkins Hospital

...alph and Barbara Alterowitz have ...llected some . . . important guideposts ...nd have illuminated them for the · ...yperson with commonsense and good ...dgment. They have presented the ...sues in a clear and informative ...anner. Where else are these issues ...ddressed, survivor to survivor, in such ...delicate and compassionate manner?

—From the Introduction by
Donald S. Coffey, Ph.D.,
Director of Urological
Research, The Johns
Hopkins Hospital

About the Authors

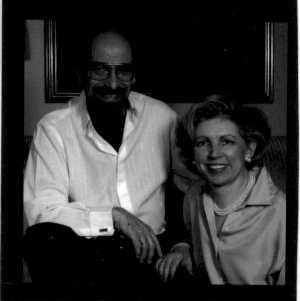

Ralph Alterowitz, the founding vice-chair and a former director of the National Prostate Cancer Coalition, is currently president of the Education Center for Prostate Cancer Patients. With 20 years of health care experience, he and his wife, Barbara, have teamed up to educate and counsel hundreds of couples on how to reestablish intimacy and loving when faced with impotence.

Ralph is president of Venture Tech Corporation, an educator and author on entrepreneurship and new ventures. Barbara is a marketing executive with a major international technology firm.

This forthright and clearly written guide, written by a [...] partner, will help men and their partners understand what affects sexual function and how to fix what is in need of repair.

> —Stephen B. Strum, M.D., prostate oncologist and director, Prostate Cancer Research Institute

A straightforward and practical book offering cancer survivors and their partners a way to begin again after cancer.

> —Jane Reese-Coulbourne, consultant and former executive vice president, National Breast Cancer Coalition

The Lovin' Ain't Over *aims a bright light at a very dark corner of the literature available to prostate patients. Existing books focus on the physical consequences of each treatment choice. This book deals most effectively with feelings and what individuals and couples can do about them. A "must read" for both survivors of, and people choosing a treatment plan for, prostate cancer.*

> —Jess Rifkind, management consultant and survivor

Excellent Advice! Unquestionably helps prostate cancer patients and survivors.

> —Charles Troshinsky, M.D., psychiatrist and survivor

[This book] should be most helpful to many couples involved with this dreadful disease. I particularly like the upbeat tone.

> —Walter Schiff, retired IBM executive and survivor

As a prostate cancer survivor who has been affected by the side effects of radiation, I believe the Alterowitzes have made a significant contribution to our problems of erectile dysfunction. The Lovin' Ain't Over *is outstanding, well-written, and should be read by all men and women.*

> —James Lewis, Jr., Ph.D., executive director, Education Center for Prostate Cancer Patients, and best-selling author of prostate cancer books.

Practical advice that applies to all relationships, not just to prostate patients. Presented candidly, but in a way that doesn't make me feel that I have to read it under the covers with a flashlight.

> —Bill Cusack, prostate cancer activist

—very hopeful, very honest, not annoyingly full of platitudes and happyspeak.

> —Donna Rifkind, book reviewer, Wall Street Journal, Baltimore Sun, and Washington Post.

THE LOVIN' AIN'T OVER™

THE LOVIN' AIN'T OVER™

The Couple's Guide to Better Sex After Prostate Disease

By
Ralph and Barbara Alterowitz

Health Education Literary Publisher
P.O. Box 948
Westbury, NY 11590
Tel: (516) 942-5000 • Fax: (516) 942-5025

Library of Congress Cataloging in Publication Data

Alterowitz, Ralph.
    The Lovin' Ain't Over : The Couple's Guide /
by Ralph and Barbara Alterowitz.
        p. cm.
    Includes bibliographical references and index.
    ISBN 1-883257-02-6
    1. Impotence Popular works. 2. Prostate—
Cancer—Complications. 3. Prostate—Cancer
Popular works. 4. Prostate—Cancer—Patients—
Sexual relationships. I. Alterowitz, Barbara,
II. Title
RC889.A46 1999   99-37186
616.6'92—dc21   CIP

Contents

Chapter 3

Chapter 6
Putting it all Together

Appendices
Appendix A
Manufacturers of Erectile Dysfunction Products

Appendix B
Resources for Erectile Dysfunction

Foreword

The topics of erection, intimacy, and love bring forward personal barriers and social taboos that almost assure that communication is dampened or denied. Just recall the last time you discussed these issues publicly or in a serious manner. The lack of thoughtful books directed to those confronting intimacy and sexual difficulties underscores the need for these issues to be addressed by patients who have experienced such problems and have sought information and solutions.

There are many approaches, and results can vary. Everyone with the same recipe cannot cook the same cake. However, even though the approaches and outcomes may vary, each couple still faces many common problems and decisions. Some guideposts help as we traverse through life's complex and sensitive paths. Certainly medical advice is central, but so are the experiences and perspectives of the patients and their partners.

Ralph and Barbara Alterowitz have collected some of these important guideposts and with common sense and good judgment have illuminated them for the layperson. They have presented the issues in a clear and informative manner. Where else are these issues addressed, survivor to survivor, in such a delicate and compassionate manner? The Alterowitzes have made a pioneering effort to illuminate this topic in a sensitive manner, and they will be thanked by the many who will say, "Thank goodness for *The Lovin' Ain't Over.*"

—Donald S. Coffey, Ph.D.
Professor and Director of
Urological Research
The Johns Hopkins Hospital

Preface

I f anyone had told us 10 years ago that we would publicly discuss intimacy and sexuality, we would have declared them crazy. But life had a surprise in store for us: Ralph developed prostate cancer. He came through it successfully and began to speak to prostate cancer support groups, initially with the idea of presenting a positive role model to newly diagnosed patients. During these conversations, many quality-of-life issues came up. Impotence was an issue people continually said they felt was not being adequately addressed, and they felt a great need to discuss it.

Armed with our own relationship as a baseline, we read books and articles, and had conversations with hundreds of prostate cancer survivors and their spouses or partners.

Fairly quickly, we found ourselves talking to support groups and at prostate cancer conferences. The interactions, questions, and comments we received confirmed that there was a great need for straight talk about this subject. For example, one couple said that after our talk they went home and talked and cried together, and then they made love for the first time in two years. Many people told us we should put our thoughts into a book.

So here you are, book in hand. You should know where we come from. This is not a clinical book. We're prostate cancer survivors (the partner is a survivor as well). We are talking not as authorities, but as people who've been there. Patient to patient, partner to partner.

This is a book from us to other couples who have survived prostate cancer. We hope it will help them restore intimacy, and rebuild, and possibly even improve, their love lives and sexuality.

We hope couples will find this book helpful as a means for opening their channels of communication. In many cases, improving your love life will require communicating in a different way than many couples are used to.

We recognize that some of this work may be difficult. In Chaim Potok's book, *In the Beginning*, David tells his students, "Be patient. You are learning a new way of understanding. . . . All beginnings are hard. . . . Especially a beginning that you make by yourself." This book focuses on understanding and building intimacy between partners. Both partners must participate in redefining their sexual relationship. Loving is a partnering activity, a way to reconnect emotionally. To successfully restore intimacy and reestablish the physical side of your relationship, each partner's participation is essential. Prostate cancer can be a wake-up call to refocus your emotional and physical relationship.

Once you have resolved to address the emotional side, there are many options to improve the physical side as well: medications, mechanical aids, herbal potions, and even some commonsense actions that can make the experience better for both partners.

Good luck and good health.

—Ralph and Barbara Alterowitz

Acknowledgments

This book could not have been written without our interaction with the hundreds of survivors and partners who participated in our "The Loving Ain't Over" sessions or talked to us individually. They asked us to write this book, contributed materials, confided in us, and provided direction and support.

Many people reviewed the manuscript. Physicians, social workers, psychiatrists, and pharmaceutical companies along with survivors and their partners made sure that the text was technically correct and that it addressed the concerns of people affected by erectile dysfunction. Dr. Richard Howe shared with us his wealth of experience as an activist, survivor, and planner and reviewer of prostate cancer research. He also scrutinized every word to greatly improve the quality. The book also received a combined critical urology, oncology, and sexual dysfunction review by Drs. Israel Barken, Arthur Burnett, and Stephen Strum, who reviewed the manuscript for accuracy, and contributed their insights on the relationship and emotional aspects. Dr. Martin Mintz of Northern Pharmacy in Baltimore added realism by clueing us into the retail pharmacy channel regarding dosages, prices, and other information.

April Becker could be called the book's godmother. She kept encouraging us, telling us how much *The Lovin' Ain't Over* was needed, and she provided significant insight from her work with couples. Laura Cline was always there for us to test ideas and concepts and to keep us from going astray.

Dr. Jim Lewis' work on treating and coping with prostate disease was very valuable. In addition, we thank him for shepherding us through the process of getting the book published.

Manufacturers of commercial therapies and aids contributed material and reviewed the accuracy of the information about their products. They helped without trying to bias the book. The companies included American MedTech, Encore, Erogenex, Harvard Scientific, Macrochem, Mission Pharmacal, NexMed, Pfizer, Pharmacia-Upjohn, Pos-T-Vac, Schwarz Pharma, TAP Pharmaceuticals, Timm Medical, VIVUS, and Zonagen.

Many other people helped with *The Lovin' Ain't Over*. Early on, Richard Leshuk prodded us to revise the structure. Many thanks to Patricia Phelan of Glanvil Enterprises, Ltd. for her diligent copy editing and to Dale Schroeder for his work on the layout.

Without Jon Zonderman, the idea of a book would not have become a reality. He stepped up to the plate to work on this project with us, even though the topic was so different from the business writing on which we usually collaborate. Jon took the raw material of our ideas and created the skeleton for the book. As in all of our projects over the past 12 years, he also added considerable clarity to our writing.

The experience of Ralph's cancer and recovery has been a spiritual journey as much as it was a medical and psychological one. We do not take life or our love for granted. They are gifts we treasure, and are thankful for.

—Barbara and Ralph Alterowitz

Introduction

It is most fortunate that *The Lovin' Ain't Over* has arrived at a time when high detection rates of prostate cancer and the rapid progress in the management of male sexual dysfunction have converged. Prostate cancer is the single most commonly diagnosed cancer and the second most common cause of cancer-related deaths in American men today. Historically, treatments for prostate cancer, including radical prostatectomy, have carried profound complications, particularly for a man's ability to achieve an erection and perform satisfactory sexual intercourse. Currently, radical prostatectomy is based on sound, anatomic techniques for preserving pelvic functions, and the potential adversities of treatment are receiving proper attention from health care professionals as well as from the general public.

Perhaps there is no better source to identify the quality-of-life issues following treatment for prostate cancer and to bring erectile dysfunction treatment to the fore than a prostate cancer survivor and his partner. Ralph and Barbara Alterowitz address these topics with a sensitivity and purpose that derives invaluably from their own personal experiences, as well as from a carefully conducted research project. They approached me to write the introduction to *The Lovin Ain't Over*, recognizing my involvement in the treatment of prostate cancer. As a urologist accomplished in the surgery of radical prostatectomy and as a specialist in erectile dysfunction management, I find this book to be a unique resource for prostate cancer patients and their partners.

The Lovin' Ain't Over captures all the considerations that men and their partners will grapple with as they contemplate the effect of prostate treatment on their sexual lives. The perspective is appropriate: sexual function pertains to humanness and love between partners, not to erection as a man's bodily function. The objective is wonderfully stated in the early passages of the text: "This book is about love in a relationship. By definition, this implies communication, sharing, and joint involvement, and of course, intimacy."

Despite its positive outlook regarding sexual health after prostate treatment, *The Lovin' Ain't Over* is more than a collection of inspirational anecdotes and reassurances. Rather, it is packed with information that enhances understanding and promotes meaningful action, enabling couples to engage in mutually satisfying lovemaking. Information is presented about the potential for gradual recovery of erectile function and the retention of other aspects of sexual function following treatment. Myths regarding male sexual prowess are dispelled. Techniques for achieving interaction and a good lovemaking experience for both partners are discussed. Finally, clinical treatment options are explored in an informative and impartial way. Consistent with multiple scientific developments in the field of erectile dysfunction that have led to new treatments, the book provides information that can be used in discussing treatments with an erectile dysfunction specialist. *The Lovin' Ain't Over* particularly reinforces the value I place on patients who take an active role in their treatment decisions and functional outcomes.

I deeply respect the insights and support provided by the Alterowitzes. They have taken a remarkable step that should serve as an example for all patients challenged with the diagnosis and treatment prospects of prostate disease.

—Arthur L. Burnett, M.D., F.A.C.S.
Associate Professor of Urology
Director, Male Sexual Health Clinic
The Johns Hopkins Hospital

NOTE TO READERS

Names of survivors and partners mentioned in
The Lovin' Ain't Over have been changed to protect
their confidentiality or are composites drawn from
our work with couples and support groups.

The Lovin' Ain't Over does not endorse any
health care product. This material is being provided
for informational purposes only.

The information contained is not intended as a
substitute for medical advice. All matters pertaining
to your mental and physical health should be
supervised by a health care provider.

The authors and publisher shall have neither
liability nor responsibility to any person or entity
with respect to any loss, damage, or injury caused
or alleged to be caused, directly or indirectly, by the
use of the information contained in this book.

Chapter 1
Impotence: An Opportunity to Regain Intimacy

Think back to when you or your partner were first diagnosed. What did you focus on when you were first told you (or your partner) had prostate cancer? If you are like us, your first thought was about survival. Then after treatment started, or the first round of therapy was over and imminent death was no longer the immediate issue, thoughts turned to: "How normal can our lives be, even if the cancer is under control? What about sex?"

Given that prostate cancer affects mostly men over 50, it is safe to say that most of us grew up at a time when sex, loving, and parts of our anatomy were not as openly discussed as they are today. When we were kids we didn't talk about loving. Boys' "locker-room" conversations were about sex.

The women, who were girls then, talked about love. Girls who "did it" were not "nice." Everyone had heard the expression, "Nice girls don't."

Despite more open discussion of sex today, the world hasn't come very far in terms of connecting sex with love.

Is it any wonder that after prostate cancer therapy, which makes men impotent to one degree or another, many or most couples do not talk about sex? They continue to treat the subject as taboo. By doing so, they build one of the biggest barriers to overcoming the problem.

Reality Hits

Even before prostate cancer therapy, most men had lost some of their sexual capability. We like to believe that we were doing almost as well sexually before prostate cancer therapy as we did when we were 20. We may have even filled out our urologist's sex questionnaire saying that we had steel-hard erections and had sex three to four times a week. But the reality is that most of us were already well into the gray zone-somewhere between our 20s' level of potency and impotence-before we were treated for prostate cancer. For some, a lifestyle of stress, smoking, and eating fatty foods had led to blockage of arteries, which does the same to the penis as to the heart. Even for those with a relatively healthy lifestyle, age-related deterioration of sexual capacity was setting in.

Sexual function had already declined due to aging, stress, and other factors.

But whatever your level of erectile function, prostate cancer therapy makes things worse in two ways. First is the psychological component. After you get the blow of the cancer diagnosis, you find out that the treatment affects your potency. Second is the physical and physiological consequences of the treatments, which highlight any underlying erectile dysfunction.

Usually, prostate cancer treatment worsens potency.

Common misconceptions can actually worsen erectile dysfunction. In his 1998 *Geriatrics* article, "Erectile dysfunction: A practical approach for primary care," Dr. Arthur Burnett, director of the Male Sexual Health Clinic at Johns Hopkins Hospital, wrote: "Erectile dysfunction carries the implication of sexual failure and is associated with anxiety, depression, marital discord, and even violence." Viagra seems to have spurred men to get help. A Pfizer study found that after Viagra became available, about 15 percent of men with erectile dysfunction went for counseling compared with 7 percent beforehand. Unfortunately, there are a lot of mistaken ideas that these men have come to believe. In the same article, Dr.

Mistaken beliefs make erectile dysfunction worse.

Burnett also notes that a number of mistaken beliefs hinder a man's ability to deal with this condition:

> ### Mistaken Beliefs
>
> - Matters relating to sexual dysfunction are taboo.
> - Loss of erections is not a common problem, and my problem is unique.
> - Erectile dysfunction is a normal part of aging.
> - Inability to achieve erections is primarily a psychological problem and not physical.
> - Treatment options are generally lacking, or are too invasive and risky to be pursued.

One major finding of an "international survey of men with prostate cancer was that too little counseling or information on treatment options and their effects on sexual function is provided to patients." (*Prostate Cancer and Prostatic Disease*, Vol. 1, No. 4, June 1998, p.182). Another study puts it bluntly: "Many men do not want counseling."

The good part is that now you are part of a community that has faced these problems, so you can talk about it, sympathize, and possibly see yourselves in the situations others describe, and you can learn from their experience.

Learn from others in the prostate cancer community.

Men's mental image of their sexual capability is often greater than "the real thing." They tend to overstate their sexual prowess. In addition, some people expect that after treatment, their erections will be as good or better than they are now. The result of treatment is usually less compatibility and, in the best case, erections that are as good as before treatment.

What do men want? An erection like in the old days? Most men over 50 have already lost some erection capability. When erections do occur, they do not last as long. It takes longer to get an erection. In addition to age, lifestyle and underlying medical conditions can have an

Fill Out Questionnaires Honestly

Some urologists have adopted the practice of using questionnaires so patients can describe their sex-life characteristics before therapy. This helps urologists to help the patient create realistic expectations. Often, men describe a level of sexual activity and performance prior to therapy that is more characteristic for a 20- to 30-year old man. In other words, the answers are often reflective not of reality, but wishful thinking. Men have the tendency to overestimate their sexual prowess.

There is a story of a man who was diagnosed with prostate cancer and told he needed surgery. He asked the doctor whether he would be able to have sex afterwards. The doctor asked him whether he was having sex now. When he said no, the doctor told him it would be the same afterward.

impact on sexual function. There may also be a "sameness" to sex with a longtime partner that reduces the excitement and pleasure.

All together, sex is not the same as it was 10, 20, or 30 years earlier.

Prostate cancer therapy often reduces sexual capability as measured by erections. But the before-and-after difference may not be as great as we imagine. This is not to say that you should not take action to overcome the problem. To the contrary, treatment for prostate cancer is a "focusing event" that allows you to redefine and refine the sexual aspects of your relationship; it puts the issue of impotence in a context of intimacy that is more complex and subtle than dealing with the cancer itself.

So we'll ask the question again: What do men want? If your answer is a happy satisfying love life for both partners, then read on. You are now a member of the brotherhood and sisterhood of surviving couples who recognize that intimacy and sexuality are essential to their relationship.

To repeat: the good news about prostate cancer treatment that causes some degree of impotence is that *it can*

Prostate cancer can serve to focus both partners on their relationship, including their sexual relationship.

force you to change your habits in your love life. It's a golden opportunity to work together toward a *much better love life for both of you.*

Relearning to make love makes your relationship new and exciting. You discover new things; you behave differently; you see sides of your partner that delight and surprise you. It's almost like having an affair with your current partner-and you don't have to feel one bit of guilt!

We are more capable than previous generations of making these changes. According to a 1973 survey (when most of us were between 25 and 45), we had already made major breaks from the sexual patterns of our parents. Here's another opportunity.

The Relationship Rut

Many couples are in a relationship rut. "If you live by the railroad tracks and a train goes by, you don't even wake up."

Many of us have gotten into a routine in our love life. The pressures of everyday life affect priorities, and for many, sex has become a lower priority. Also, at the age when you are likely to get prostate cancer, sex hormones don't drive men the way they used to. You may not get "turned on" by your partner as much anymore, and living with her (or him) may have become routine. The situation is what psychologists call "habituation." Patricia Love, Ed.D., author of *Hot Monogamy* (Plume, 1995), has a colorful way of putting it: "If you live by the railroad tracks and a train goes by, you don't even wake up." As one survivor's wife put it: "A lot of things fall by the wayside when you're married awhile."

Judith Wallerstein, in her book *The Good Marriage: How and Why Love Lasts* (Houghton Mifflin, 1995), says "a good sex life, however the couple defines that, is at the heart of a good marriage." Of the nine fundamental characteristics of a good marriage, she found that sexual love is sixth. "This is the domain where intimacy is renewed, and the excitement that first drew the couple together is kept alive. . . . There is no better antidote to the pressures of living than a loving sex life."

Rather than a door closing, impotence problems after prostate cancer therapy can be a door opening to a new experience that enriches your relationship. Opening yourself to a new perspective of what loving is all about can offer both of you opportunities for broader communication and for seeing ways for altering your respective styles of loving. Introducing newness into your lovemaking can energize you and increase your enthusiasm. In this book, we will look at some of the emotional and anatomical factors that bear on this.

This book is about love in a relationship. By definition, that means we must talk about communication, sharing, joint involvement, and of course, intimacy.

Gail Sheehy defines the capacity for intimacy as "the art of giving to another while still maintaining a lively sense of self." In other words, for each of us, our capacity for intimacy is being able to be me, you, and us. Each partner has to express his or her own personality, needs, and desires during lovemaking, while simultaneously being thoughtful about the needs of his or her partner.

The basic premise for this entire discussion is: *You can have a loving and satisfying sexual relationship without having an erection.* We'll give you some tips on aids for getting an erection, but we urge you not to focus on the erection-you'll both have much more fun and satisfaction with the experience.

Erections are important, but shouldn't be the sole focus.

Impotence: An Opportunity to Regain Intimacy

Key Points

- Sexuality is an essential aspect of intimacy, and intimacy is the foundation of a loving relationship.
- Men with erectile dysfunction usually still have sexual desire and can have a satisfying love life.
- Loving is more than intercourse.
- There is a broad range of loving activities to compensate for varying degrees of impotence.
- Both partners must work together to achieve a mutually satisfying experience.

Chapter 2
Facts About Impotence

We use the two terms *impotence* and *erectile dysfunction (ED)* interchangeably. Impotence is a man's inability to obtain and maintain an erection sufficient for intercourse. Unfortunately, people tend to think of impotence as if it indicates a total and irrevocable condition. In reality, there are different levels of erectile dysfunction, or impotence, and many of them can be addressed.

With impotence becoming a more public topic, estimates have begun appearing in health reports that about 18 to 30 million (the Mayo Clinic estimates 30 to 35 million) American men have problems with erections and suffer varying degrees of impotence from physical causes. Actually, 10 percent of all men have problems at age 30, and it increases from there. By the time men are in their 50s and 60s, about half have experienced significant erectile dysfunction.

Ten percent of 30-year-old men have difficulty attaining and maintaining erections; about half of the men 60 or older have erection problems.

Causes of Erectile Dysfunction

Erectile function is affected by some things men have control over and by other things men have no control over.

In addition to prostate cancer therapy, erectile dysfunction can be caused by accident, injury, or disease. In some instances, even medications can cause or worsen erectile dysfunction.

About a dozen chronic diseases cause varying degrees of impotence. Diabetes is responsible for about 40 percent of cases, vascular and heart disease for about 30 percent, radical surgery for about 13 percent, spinal injury for about 8 percent, and endocrine disorders for about 6 percent. Some of these diseases are made worse by lifestyle, and all are complicated by the effects of aging.

There are three major "lifestyle" causes of erectile dysfunction.

Chronic illness is responsible for over 70 percent of impotence cases.

- **Alcohol**—People talk of going out to eat and drink and then making love. Alcohol is seen as "loosening people up" and making them more receptive about engaging in sex. While a little alcohol, a glass of wine or a beer, can decrease anxiety and inhibition, more than this acts as a sedative. It makes people sleepy and less able to actively participate. In many men, it has a negative effect on the ability to have an erection and an orgasm.

- **Street and Prescription Drugs**—A range of prescription drugs available today lessens the ability and the energy to make love. Some drugs, both prescription and street drugs, increase desire and a sense of sensuality, but *decrease* erectile function.

- **Smoking**—Research has increasingly shown the direct cause-and-effect relationship between smoking and erectile dysfunction. Nicotine directly interferes with nerve pathways and circulation, which decreases a man's ability to have good erections. Smoking clogs up the small blood vessels in the penis as well as in the heart. Obviously, if the blood vessels are clogged, erections cannot occur.

Alcohol, drugs and smoking are the three major lifestyle factors that cause erectile dysfunction.

Table 2–1, taken from the *Handbook of Sexual Dysfunction,* shows medications with negative effects on desire (libido) and potency. These are medications prescribed to cope with and control cardiovascular

11

Table 2-1. Pharmacological Agents Known to Cause Sexual Dysfunction

Condition	Agents	Description/Comments
Impotence	Atenolol (Tenormin)	impotence
	Amitriptyline (Elavil)	impotence, loss of libido
	Chlorthalidone (Hygroton)	impotence, decreased libido
	Cimetidine (Tagamet)	impotence, decreased libido
	Clofibrate (Atromid)	impotence, decreased libido
	Diazepam (Valium)	difficult erection, no orgasm in women
	Digoxin (Lanoxin)	impotence, decreased libido
	Disulfiram (Antabuse)	impotence
	Famotidine (Pepcid)	impotence
	Gemfibrozil (Lopid)	impotence, loss of libido
	Hydralazine (Apresoline)	impotence, priapism
	Indapamide (Lozol)	impotence, decreased libido
	Indomethacin (Indocin)	impotence, decreased libido
	Labetalol (Trandate)	impotence, decreased libido
	Leuprolide (Lupron)	impotence
	Lithium (Lithobid)	impotence, decreased libido
	Metoclopramide (Reglan)	impotence, decreased libido
	Metoprolol (Lopressor)	impotence
	Mexiletine (Mexitil)	impotence, decreased libido
	Naproxen (Naprosyn)	impotence, no ejaculation
	Omeprazole (Prilosec)	painful nocturnal erection
	Phenytoin (Dilantin)	impotence, decreased libido
	Primidone (Mysoline)	impotence, decreased libido
	Propanolol (Inderal)	impotence, decreased libido
	Ranitidine (Zantac)	impotence, decreased libido
	Spironolactone (Aldactone)	impotence, decreased libido
	Thiazide (Diuretics)	impotence, decreased libido
	Verapamil (Calan)	impotence
Decreased/Delayed Libido/Orgasm	Alprazolam (Xanax)	decreased libido, delayed orgasm
	Amiodarone (Cordarone)	decreased libido
	Amphetamine	no orgasm (men and women)
	Desipramine (Norpramin)	painful orgasm
	Fluoxetine (Prozac)	no orgasm, decreased libido
	Lorazepam (Ativan)	loss of libido
	Methyldopa (Aldomet)	decreased libido and orgasm
	Radiation therapy	decreased libido, low ejaculatory volume
Priapism	Psychotropic agents (Chlorpromazine)	
	Antihypertensives (Hydralazine, Prazosin)	
	Antidepressant (Trazodone)	
	Vasoactive agents (Papaverine, PGE1)	

problems such as hypertension and angina, anxiety, depression, psychosis, and other conditions.

If you suspect that a prescription drug is causing impotence, ask your doctor if there is an alternative medication that may not have this effect. If you are taking street drugs, stop immediately. If you are dependent on a drug, seek help if you want to preserve your love life.

Sex and Getting Older

What is a "Normal" Sex Life?

Many people try to measure and quantify everything, including how often they make love. It seems like many of us are searching for the holy grail in sex. But what is "normal"? In November 1998, the *New York Times* said: "Most couples consider good sex vital to a marriage's success, but have sex about once a week, for an average of 39 minutes." (While writing this section, we were listening to Ravel's "Bolero,"-considered a very erotic piece of music. Unfortunately, it has to be played three times to accompany the average American loving because it's only 13 minutes long.)

A survey showed that "Americans fall into three groups. One third have sex twice a week or more, one third just a few times a month, and the last one third have sex a few times a year or not at all."

In 1973, couples who then were 35 to 45 years old (today's 60 to 70-year-olds) had sex 99 times a year, almost twice weekly. But, since this number is the median, half of the couples were above and half were below.

Even the Viagra market forecasters could not decide what "normal" is. They prepared revenue forecasts based on a man using the pill from twice a month to as much as twice a week. The bottom line is:

> *Normal for you and your partner is whatever gives you both pleasure. Both partners need to agree on how often they should make love to make their life satisfying.*

How often is normal for you? Whatever you and your partner agree on.

"It's Over"—or Is It?

While we're talking about the issue of what's normal, it *is* normal to be interested in sex throughout your life. Men and women can, and many think should, remain sexually active throughout their entire lives. No one has to apologize for an interest in sex.

Some people believe that sex is only for the young and that older people are expected to lose their desire for sex and their ability to "perform." One doctor told us that his father asked him for a prescription for Viagra, but asked that he have another doctor in the practice sign the prescription because "your mother doesn't want you to know that we are still having sex."

Millions of men have given up on lovemaking because of their erection problems. In our prostate cancer community, one study found that the level of expressed "sexual interest" dropped by half after treatment. Actual sexual activity dropped by almost two-thirds as measured by the "frequency of . . . passionate kissing, sexually touching and sexual intercourse" (*Prostate Cancer and Prostatic Diseases*, June 1998).

The physical problems men have are worsened by the "mind trips" they take. They create excuses such as:

"I'm not interested anymore."

"I've got other things to do."

"I'm getting too old."

"There is nothing I can do about it."

"What's the point? It won't work anyway."

The fact is, men can continue to have a strong sex drive even if they have erectile dysfunction. It is possible to have good loving for the rest of your life regardless of age, whether you have erectile dysfunction or not. Many men with erectile dysfunction still have some erectile capability. And even without intercourse, you can still have a good love life. It is not necessary to have an erection for either partner to have an orgasm.

With aging, arousal takes longer for a number of reasons. This can be seen as a blessing in disguise because it

Even without intercourse, you can still have a good love life.

14

can make loving much better. In general, women take longer to become aroused. Therefore, if a man takes longer as well, his partner may be aroused or nearly there by the time he is. This synchronicity of arousal can help both parties to experience the same pleasure and can remove one of the main complaints younger women have about their love life.

Could She Possibly be Interested?

Many men assume their partners are not interested in sex because the partner has not initiated it or talked about it in a while. Assuming, rather than asking, is a bad thing in a relationship. There may be a variety of reasons why she has not brought it up:

- She may be interested, but thinks that he is not.

- She may be interested and sense that he is too, but, knowing about (or guessing about) the impotence problem, she does not want to "put him on the spot."

- She may truly not be interested.

You'll never know unless you talk about it.

It becomes a big job for a couple to counteract the man's bruised ego when he has erection problems.

You must remember that *any problem that affects one person in a relationship affects the other person as well.*

When lack of physical intimacy becomes an issue for a couple, both of them-not the man alone-may become fixated on it. They think about it when they hear someone talk about love, about sex, or even watch a movie with a love scene. It affects all parts of both the man's and the woman's lives. They may even avoid anything that could bring it up, ultimately leading both partners to enter a "conspiracy of silence."

A woman may unwittingly give the impression that she's not interested in sex if she enters into a conspiracy of silence with her partner. Being aware of his erectile dysfunction, she may not want to bring it up because

You don't need an erection for either partner to have an orgasm.

Partners may create a "conspiracy of silence" when they have sexual problems.

A happy love life depends on open communication—and that includes talking about the difficult things.

she's afraid to hurt him. She assumes that the man will bring it up when he feels like it. But men, especially those of the born-before-WWII generation, were not raised to talk about things that could embarrass them. In his autobiography, Joseph Heller (of *Catch-22* fame) describes the communications psychology of pre-WWII men. He says, "It would have been hard to tell if our health hadn't been good, since no one in our family made a fashion of ailments or talked much about the distress they brought." We think he sums it up beautifully: "But not only did we not complain much in my family, we didn't talk much about anything deeply felt." The last thing men want to do is raise a problem where they have something at stake, something to risk, when they do not know how to handle it.

If you want to have a happy love life, one of you will have to bring the subject up in a loving way. The problem does not go away or get better if you don't talk about it. It becomes a barrier. You've got to open up and ask the question, "If we can't make love the way we used to, how else can we please each other?" And don't forget to mention what would make you happy. Those conversations, and the resulting actions, open up the channel of communication between you-and that's the basis for intimacy.

Sex and the Older Woman

Another myth related to sex and the older person is that women aren't interested in sex and loving as they get older. That is true for some women, but studies have shown that many women over 50 become increasingly more interested in sex because the danger of pregnancy is reduced or gone, and there are fewer family-raising pressures in their lives.

A woman whose partner introduced her to lubricants at age 60 says she "can't get enough of it (sex)." Again, the only way to find out if your partner is interested is to talk with her.

Prostate Cancer Treatment Effects: What's the Truth?

Am I the Only One With a Problem?

Survivors assume, "I'm the only one who has a problem. Everyone else came out of therapy OK." The truth is that 70 to 90 percent of prostate cancer survivors have erectile dysfunction *for some time, or permanently.*

Leslie Shover, Ph.D., of the Cleveland Clinic Foundation, reported that "the prevalence of sexual problems may be as high as . . . 70 percent in prostate cancer survivors." (*Journal of the National Cancer Institute* Vol. 90, No. 8, April 15, 1998, p. 566). Dr. Shover goes on to note that "Problems faced by survivors include loss of desire, erectile dysfunction, painful intercourse, and difficulty reaching orgasm."

For surgery patients, the statistics are that as many as 90 percent will have erectile dysfunction immediately following treatment. Recovery varies widely. One prominent medical center (known for prostate surgery) estimates that about 40 percent of their surgery patients will recover "full function" within six months and about 60 to 70 percent will recover within 18 months. However, every procedure results in some loss of erectile capability. Even if nerves are not cut during surgery, some nerves are damaged.

A relatively high potency-recovery rate may be expected with surgical excellence. This is illustrated by one study citing low recovery rates following surgery by 30 doctors with varying levels of training and experience. By contrast, highly skilled surgeons quote recovery rates in the 60 to 70 percent range. Recovery for younger men is higher than for older men. The skill of the surgeon is an important factor in recovering potency, but not the only one.

Nerves are also damaged during radiation. Where radiation therapy is concerned, erectile dysfunction appears to be delayed according to a recent paper in a cancer journal. About 20 to 30 percent of radiation patients have erectile dysfunction right after therapy.

70 to 90 percent of prostate cancer survivors have erectile dysfunction for some time, or permanently.

For surgery patients, the skill of the doctor is an important factor in recovering potency, but not the only one.

Five years after radiation therapy, survivors have about the same level of erectile dysfunction as surgery patients.

Maybe there is a gap between what doctors consider "full function" and what patients perceive as "good."

18

Radiation damages the small blood vessels supplying the pelvic region. This leads to fibrosis (scarring that causes toughening) of these small blood vessels. The scarring process builds on itself by interfering with nutrients, blood flow, and oxygenation. In time, the tissue goes from soft to leathery.

As a result, five years after radiation therapy, survivors have about the same level of erectile dysfunction as do surgery patients. Although potency is higher in the near term compared with surgery, ultimately the level of impotence resulting from radiation may be comparable to that resulting from surgery.

Nerve-Sparing Operations: The Miracle Treatment?

Another bit of prostate cancer mythology is this: After a nerve-sparing operation the man has the same level of potency as he had before the surgery. We all wish it were true, but it's usually not.

The nerves responsible for erections run alongside the prostate, not through it. Because nerves run along blood vessels, surgeons can see the nerve-blood vessel (neurovascular) bundles. Although nerves are not visible to the naked eye, surgeons generally know the surgical landmarks. Therefore it's possible to spare these areas. However, even when the neurovascular bundles are spared, the nerves are traumatized, and smaller ones are not seen and cut.

In 1997, the FDA approved a nerve-locating tool, the CaverMap Surgical Aid. UroMed, the manufacturer, said that the patented technology helps surgeons map microscopic cavernous nerves. The system is currently being used at the Johns Hopkins University and other centers of excellence. While the device is still imprecise, more precise technologies may come along now that a breakthrough has been made.

We know of a support group formed by a number of survivors who where operated on by a prominent surgeon noted for his nerve-sparing surgical technique. They shared their experiences and tracked how everyone fared. They found that although the doctor's statistics were very good, almost everyone experienced significant erectile dysfunction. Maybe there is a gap between what doctors consider "full function" and what patients perceive as "good."

Is Potency Known Immediately After Surgery?

Potency is rarely known immediately after treatment. Any therapy is a shock to the system. After surgery, it may take two years (and sometimes longer) to recover and to find out how potent you really are, although some medical centers quote shorter times. This has been confirmed by several survivors, but most survivors tell us that no one ever told them this in advance.

So if you recently had treatment and are now experiencing impotence, there is a possibility that your erectile function will improve over time, especially if you immediately begin manual stimulation (see Chapter 4) and various other techniques (see Chapter 5).

Potency may take two to three years to return.

Does Hormone Treatment Destroy Desire and Potency?

With complete hormonal blockade, desire and potency will be minimal. However, current research on monotherapy with non-steroidal antiandrogens such as "flutamide and nilutamide show that libido and potency may be retained in 70–80% of patients." (*Prostate Cancer and Prostatic Disease*, Vol. 1, No. 4, June 1998, p. 183).

Can Sex Stimulate Cancer, or Can I Transmit Cancer to My Partner Through Sex?

A recent study reported that some patients decide not to pursue lovemaking because of concerns related to the disease itself. These concerns include a belief that sex will stimulate the cancer, and possibly transmit the cancer to their partners. Both of these are absolutely false.

Effects of Treatment for Benign Prostatic Hyperplasia (BPH)

Patients with benign prostatic hyperplasia (BPH), a non-cancerous enlargement of the prostate with resulting bladder outflow obstruction and lower urinary tract symptoms, can receive a treatment called transurethral resection of the prostate (TURP). Although providing the highest likelihood of relief of both prostatic symptoms and urinary flow obstruction, surgical intervention for BPH with procedures such as TURP can have a significant impact on the patient's sexual function. Two main symptoms affect sexuality: First, erectile dysfunction, with rates reported as high as 14%. The second effect is retrograde ejaculation, which means that the ejaculate flows back into the body instead of flowing out of the penis. This affects 68% of TURP patients.

General Questions and Answers About Impotence

Do I Need an Erection In Order to Have an Orgasm?

An impotent man can have an orgasm. *An erection is not needed for an orgasm.* The facts are:

- Men without prostates do have orgasms and simulated ejaculations. Pelvic muscles contract, so that you feel as if you had an ejaculation. As we will discuss in Chapter 3, different sets of nerves are responsible for erections and orgasms, so it is possible to have an orgasm when the penis is limp.

  Without a prostate, these orgasms are not accompanied by ejaculate, even if it feels as if you had one. Some men may have a small amount of ejaculate, but most men will have a dry orgasm. Nevertheless, the orgasm feels the same as with ejaculate. Some men get upset when there is no ejaculate. One such man told us, "Now I know I'm not a man." But the focus should be on the sensation, not the ejaculation.

- Men can have sensations and release during orgasm without an erection similar to those they had with an erection.

- Orchiectomy patients (those who have had their testes removed) can have orgasms. These patients have achieved erections watching pornographic movies. Even orchiectomy patients in their 80s have had "wet dreams." Some of these men have also had erections after taking medications. The key to having erections and orgasms is that these men have known desire and experienced orgasms, thus proving again that sex is in the mind.

Can My Partner Have an Orgasm if I Don't Have an Erection?

A woman does not need penetration to have an orgasm.

Men and women are lucky because the organ that causes a woman's orgasm is on the outside. There are many ways for a woman to experience pleasure and to achieve an orgasm, even with a partner who has no erection at all. Stimulation of the clitoris does not require an erection. (Read more about this in Chapter 4 under "Loving Is A Partnering Activity.")

Orgasm = Satisfaction?

Many men believe that an orgasm is needed for a satisfying sexual experience.

Most women know this is not true. Many men have never given themselves a chance to find this out.

An orgasm is a wonderful benefit but it does not have to be the goal of lovemaking.

Does Size Matter?

Even if they don't have erectile dysfunction, some surgery patients find that they've lost an inch of penis length or more through the treatment. This ties right in with a deep-seated anxiety: men assume that a woman's love for them is related to the size of their sexual organ.

Size has little to do with the ability to give pleasure.

21

Masters and Johnson disproved this myth in the 1960s. A more accurate statement is that the quality of the lovemaking experience is an important part of keeping a relationship vibrant and vital.

Although men know intellectually that their wives or partners don't love them for their "size," they have a lot of anxiety related to this issue. As a couple goes through the difficult time after diagnosis and treatment, it's very important for the woman to keep telling the patient why she loves him, and what she loves about the relationship. Don't leave out what you love about the physical relationship-most of its quality is not related to his "size" anyway!

While size can be a visual stimulant for a woman, most women are much more affected by touch than by visual factors. And let's face it: We didn't marry an "erection machine"-we married a man with whom we wanted to spend our lives because he was a great guy. Maybe a part of that was that he was a great lover. And he can still be a great lover, even without a giant erection! In fact, even without any erection at all.

Facts About Impotence

Key Points

- Many physical factors cause impotence, but this need not prevent us from having a good love life.

- You can't control accidents, disease, or injuries, but you can keep alcohol, drugs, and smoking from ruining your sex life.

- There is no prescribed "normal frequency" for lovemaking —you and your partner define "normal."

- Erectile dysfunction is widespread. It's not a "yes or no" condition—there is a continuum of potency.

- You can have good loving, even with erectile dysfunction.

- Men's delay in arousal as they get older brings them more in tune with women.

- It's okay, normal, and healthy to make love as you get older. Loving and sex are a measure of the health of a marriage and the health of each partner.

- One of you must bring up the issues of impotence and alternative ways to please each other in a loving way that opens up communication between you. Entering into a "conspiracy of silence" is destructive to your relationship and isolates partners from each other.

- Sometimes it takes more than two years to recover potency after prostate cancer treatment.

- Men and women can have orgasms without erections.

- Don't worry about the size of your penis.

Chapter 3
Arousal

By the time men and women are in their late 50s and 60s, they are better matched sexually.

S timulation, arousal, excitement-whatever you want to call it, you *need* it if you are going to make love. It makes some medications work better, and *the majority of medications only work if you are aroused.*

Aging and prostate cancer therapy can really contribute to compatible loving. Early in our lives, women are sexually receptive but do not achieve orgasm as quickly as men because women have a lot of estrogen, which tempers the effect of their testosterone. The high level of testosterone in young men gives them their sex drive, and drives them to quick orgasms.

As women grow older, their estrogen levels decrease so their testosterone has a greater effect, and they become aroused and achieve orgasm more readily. By the time men and women are in their late 50s and 60s, they are better matched sexually. Men take longer to achieve orgasm and get more pleasure out of foreplay, and women are quicker to achieve orgasm.

But many women become turned off-or are not interested in sex-because their partners don't romance them, court them, or really "make love" to them. According to an 1873 quote in the *Oxford Universal Dictionary,* "Romance goes out of a man's head when the hair gets gray." What we know today is that romance is really not a matter of age, but it tends to fall by the wayside when you get so used to each other that every aspect of the relationship becomes routine. Falling into a routine is like casting a spell on love. Nobody is interested in a mechanical act.

Falling into a routine is like casting a spell on love.

Generally, men tend to be more oriented toward the "sex" part (penetration) and women toward the "loving" part (touching and experiencing tenderness). But the two aren't really that far apart. Loving starts with caring and desire. Desire means saying "I want you" in so many ways. Both men and women want to get that message from their partner. What begins with tenderness, caressing, and kissing may evolve into sex, or may be cherished by itself. Sex without loving and tenderness is a mechanical act. One of the women we talked to told her husband, "I want you to come near me but not always to come."

The occurrence of impotence is a chance for a couple to get more in tune with each other. It's a golden opportunity to improve the relationship. We've received comments from several women who say loving and sex have become better since prostate therapy. The man's delay in arousal brings his timing in sync with the woman's. In addition, many men come to grips with reduced erections, and take the time to enjoy the touching and other activities that used to be called foreplay. Putting more emphasis on sensual touching can greatly increase arousal and satisfaction for both partners.

Impotence can improve the relationship and lovemaking.

Creating the Mood

Getting aroused is about getting into a mood, just as you would to paint, write, or make beautiful music. We're reminded of the time we saw Isaac Stern in a class of Japanese children who had studied the Suzuki method of playing the violin. After one girl played a piece for him in a kind of automatic, "technical" fashion, he asked her to think about the piece in a certain way. He created the picture of the mood, of the feeling. She played the piece again, this time with caring, sensitivity, and tenderness. The difference between her first and second recital is the same as the difference between sex as a mechanical act and true loving.

There is a strong interplay between a couple's relationship and their physiology-their body's functions. Physiology is affected when the relationship is bad, or when either partner is insecure in physical intimacy. For

There is a strong interplay between a couple's relationship and their physiology—their body's functions.

If a man worries about having an erection, he is less likely to get one.

Seduction and a romantic environment increase arousal and make loving more exciting.

example, if a man is afraid that he cannot have an erection, he is much less likely to get one. Sex therapists say that the presence of sex indicates a healthy relationship. Without sex, many couples are in stress as measured by chemical levels. Sex lubricates a relationship.

As men get older, erections do not come easily or quickly, and certainly not by being willed. Focusing on performance is counterproductive because you are putting pressure on yourself. The greater the anxiety over whether you can have an erection, the greater the likelihood that you will not have it, even with medication. Chronic anxiety can override the effects of most medications.

For a man with erectile dysfunction, erections must be desired. However, they only arise with positive stimuli that trigger enzymes and neurological responses, creating arousal.

Part of arousal comes from a feeling of seduction and romance. Romance should be the cocoon you spin for your life, but especially whenever you want to make love. It is a state of being. It may include flowers, dinner, music, conversation, touching, and holding, whatever fits your style-but the most important thing is to make your partner feel loved and desired. Remember that your most important sexual organ is your brain! Sophia Loren was right on when she said "After all, sexiness is all mental. It starts here (pointing to her head) and then goes somewhere else. . . ."

Create the environment of love/romance/seduction. Since more men than woman seem to be "romance-impaired", we decided to include a few suggestions from your fellow men which will improve your romance quotient:

• Call your significant other from an outside phone.

  "Hon, how about dinner and dancing? You know, I would like you to wear that blue outfit I like"

  "I'm coming home a little earlier; would you like to slip into. . . ?"

- Put a gift in a little package, give it to the maitre d' and ask him to have the waiter serve on a serving plate with a cover.

- When she goes to the powder room, slip a note under her plate, asking her if she's got plans after dinner.

- When she goes out, have her favorite cocktail or wine waiting for her when she comes home.

- Write her a love letter.

- Get her favorite flowers. If you don't know what her favorite kind is, at least get her flowers.

- Go to the local amusement park, take a ride on the carousel, have an ice cream, and be the young lovers you are at heart.

The idea is to create an environment that can be conducive and suggestive so that you're both sending each other signals of desire.

Be romantic. Treat her like the woman you fell for.

- make her feel desirable.

- make her feel special.

- Say nice things to your lover, even if she knows you're stretching it.

Learning about Your Own Anatomy — and about Each Other's Anatomy

First, here's a brief outline about how erections happen. An erection occurs when the brain sends a signal down the spinal cord and through the nerves that sweep

Three different sets of nerves control erections, orgasms, and getting pleasure from touch.

down into the pelvis. The arteries that carry blood into the penis receive a signal from the nervous system to expand. The nerves that allow a man to feel pleasure when he is touched run in a different path from the nerves that control blood flow.

Orgasms are controlled by a third set of nerves, which runs higher up in a man's trunk. They are also controlled by the nerves that carry pleasure signals. These nerves cause the muscles around the penis to squeeze in rhythm and send messages of pleasure to the man's brain.

Thus, even if nerve damage or blocked arteries prevent a man from getting natural erections, he can almost always feel pleasure from being touched. He can also still reach orgasm.

After surgery or other therapies, sensitivity in the man's genital area is usually different. Before surgery, many or most areas in the genital area were sensitive for arousal. During surgery and radiation, nerves are cut or otherwise damaged. A man may suddenly find new points of sensitivity that he didn't even know or think about before. For example, after surgery some men feel a higher sense of arousal in the anal area than in the pubic area. This area was sensitive before treatment, but the sensitivity in the pubic area was usually so great that it overshadowed the response in the anal region. Similarly, the orgasm sensation may be felt in different areas.

Therefore, you need to explore and find out what areas are sensitive and give you pleasure, and discuss it with your partner. Sometimes you need to "negotiate" a little since the partner may not enjoy touching you in a newly sensitive area. Then you have to find alternatives. What you do in loving should give both of you pleasure.

Getting Prepared

Part of keeping the old magic going is to avoid turn-offs. Some of these actions may always have been part of your "routine." For example, shower and/or wash up completely before sex or an outing that could lead to sex.

If you've eaten ethnic foods noted for garlic, onions, curries, or other strong ingredients, deal with that before getting close to each other.

If your beard grows fast and you haven't shaved recently, your partner may not be too thrilled when you rake your bristles across her tender skin.

Prostate cancer also necessitates some additional preparations. The man should void before activity begins. Prostate surgery survivors have only one sphincter. Therefore they are more likely to have urinary leaks-stress incontinence-than will men who have had radiation. Have a towel or some tissues handy, and don't hesitate to use them if you leak. Prompt use will avoid unpleasantness. It can be no more than a "quick dab" and will not interfere. Let's face it, these annoyances will be there. The question is, do you manage them or do you let them control you and interfere with the enjoyment both of you can have?

As we get older, the genital organs have less natural lubrication. In one study, about 60 percent of women reported discomfort during sexual intercourse, vaginal dryness, and other physical symptoms that are now referred to as Female Sexual Arousal Disorder.

It's a good idea to lubricate the vagina as well as the penis. KY Jelly and Astroglide are two of the better lubricants. Body heat tends to liquefy Astroglide, which is also more natural-feeling. And then, of course, there is the most natural of all lubricants, saliva.

Some couples like to have their partners use perfume or cologne. There's nothing wrong with the man smelling good. Women like men to use cologne as much as men like women to use perfume. Make sure the partner likes the scent, and use just enough that it smells nice and not so much that either one of you wants to escape.

Some people get what's known as coital headaches from intercourse. Sex causes blood pressure to build in many places, including your head. Viagra has also been known to cause headaches. Taking an aspirin may eliminate the headache, or at least reduce it. Again, this is not a recommendation, just something you may want to explore with your doctor.

Handle urinary leaks during sex with a towel or tissues.

Use lubricants to replace natural moisture.

Touching is key to becoming aroused.

Touchpoints

Touchpoints are areas of the body that partners may find sensitive and desirable to explore. You can kiss, caress softly and gently, and squeeze touchpoints. Some women get excited with hard squeezes, but many get turned off. As we have said before, you need to communicate. Don't counteract all your stage setting and preparations by doing something that turns your partner off.

Since the touching sensation is key to becoming aroused, we have listed some body areas that people may find sensitive. We are not coming at this from the perspective of books that focus on "sexual acupressure," but merely noting some areas that could help increase the stimulation for both partners.

- Women may like men to touch or kiss them in the following places:

  - Face: Many women like a man to gently run his fingers across their face and to kiss their face and eyes. Touching the crown of her head or running your fingers through her hair can also be extremely erotic.

  - Neck: Gentle kisses or touches on the neck. The back of the neck at the base of the skull is very sensitive to light touches.

  - Hands: If you are sitting watching a movie or talking with one another, gently touching the back of her hand could help in relaxing her and getting her into the right mood. Stroking the palm has always been considered an invitation, and for good reason!

  - Earlobes: The earlobes are sensitive, probably because the blood flow is strong.

  - Feet: When she's resting with her feet on your lap, play with her toes or caress her legs.

- Buttocks: Though not one of the most sensitive areas, many people find buttock-touching to be a "turn-on."

- Breasts: The sides of the breasts are very sensitive because of the nerve endings there. Unfortunately, many men think that squeezing breasts hard will throw the partner into rapturous delight. Just imagine she was doing the same to your testicles, and you get an approximate idea about the level of enthusiasm this will generate in most women.

- You need to know your partner to know how much caressing of the nipples is desired. Some women find their nipple areas so sensitive that they are easily irritated. Yet other women find it one of the most sensitive and desirable areas that they like touched. The key point is, there are many nerve endings, and the woman needs to tell the man what is pleasurable and what is painful. Pinching and hard squeezing are usually off-limits.

- And of course, the genital area, especially the clitoris, is very sensitive. Running your fingers from the surrounding area to the pubic area and the thighs can increase arousal.

- The whole body: There is nothing more seductive than the feeling that your lover wants to explore every inch of your body. Slow touching and caressing can be extremely arousing.

- Areas that men like touched include:

  - Most of the areas discussed above for women.

  - Head of the penis: The head is particularly sensitive. Stroking the side and across the top can arouse a man. Unfortunately, extensive rubbing of the very tip can irritate the penis, much as with the woman's nipple and clitoris.

  - Scrotum around the testes: Caressing the scrotum can be very pleasurable for the woman and the man, but beware of squeezing. Squeezing the testes produces great pain, guaranteed to turn the man into a contortionist.

- Behind the penis almost between the legs (perineal area).

- Breasts: Most men have not experimented enough to know whether their breasts are sensitive. Many men are extremely sensitive to touching in the nipple area.

- Chest: Many men like women to run their hands over their chests. It makes them feel manly and desirable. Men have a need to feel desirable and appreciated as a man.

What's Your Style?

Another thing that helps in arousing your lover's passion is to know which of the senses is his or her primary "driver" for arousal. Of course, all senses play together, but as Susan Rako, M.D., author of *The Hormones of Desire* says, *"We each have a dominant sense-sight (visual), sound (auditory), or touch (kinesthetic). Play to your partner's dominant sensory preference and you trip the wire that makes sex sizzle."*

More women are stimulated by touch than by sight.

Generally, women are more touch-oriented, and men more visually oriented. The size of the man's sexual organ is primarily a visual stimulant for a woman, and since more women are stimulated by touch than by sight, those male worries about size can just fall away. How much pleasure a woman gets from the size of a man's penis depends on the size of her vaginal canal. A man who is "too big" for a woman can actually hurt her during intercourse in certain positions, so all those stories about women wanting men as large as possible are typical testosterone-overload myths.

Giving and Receiving

Don't get frantic thinking that both partners must always be active at the same time. It's perfectly okay for one of you to lay back and enjoy while the other is doing all the touching. Later, or another time, you'll reverse roles. And don't forget that touching can be just as pleasurable as being touched.

Both partners need to get used to the idea of taking turns pleasing each other. It's OK to ask your partner to do something you would enjoy, and reciprocate later.

Visualization

Visualization is a technique that has worked for people in many fields, from business presentations to sports. It's imagining yourself in a positive situation. You can use visualization to improve your lovemaking, too.

Set aside 20 minutes when you are not likely to be disturbed. Some people find it worthwhile to tell their partners they are doing visualization. This shows the partner that you are really interested. Then imagine yourself and your partner in the most positive, loving, exciting, and mutually satisfying lovemaking. Or, if there were some rough spots the last time you made love, imagine how it could be handled better and what you could do if it happened again. If you think of any problems, these might be issues that you discuss beforehand. Discussing the problems will encourage your partner to tell you about concerns she or he may have. You might also try a joint visualization, a shared fantasy about being with each other.

There are many books about visualization. The purpose here is merely to mention a technique that could help.

Visualization can enhance your lovemaking.

Handling Differences

In the psychological literature, resolving differences might be called "conflict resolution." Differences in the partners' likes and dislikes in loving can be very tricky and sometimes explosive. Our culture, upbringing, religion, and personalities dictate what you like and what you will accept. There may be differences between you and your partner regardless of how long the two of you have been together. These differences will remain there regardless of your joint efforts. They may be minimized, but they will still be there.

The only way to avoid huge battles, big "mads," and the cessation of loving is to work out a way of handling them. If both of you are aware of your respective differences, the best thing is to discuss them before you get to the loving activities. You can discuss whether or not to engage in certain behaviors, or how to modify them so they can be accepted. There is no right or wrong answer or solution. It is purely a matter of your reactions, what you want, how to please each other, and mutual satisfaction. This same approach can be applied to differences in other areas of life as well.

Regardless of whether you're rich or poor, thin or heavy, young or old, or impotent or potent, you can be a great lover! What it takes is sincere interest, commitment, and desire from both partners.

Arousal

Key Points

- The three key words for romantic and sexual health: *Communicate, communicate, communicate!*

- You can have a lot of loving without a lot of sex. A loving relationship involves many different ways to be sexually active.

- Each couple is different. Find out what makes both of you happy.

- Your most important sexual organ is "between the ears."

- Attitude is critical: Couples who are partners see love not as an exotic destination, but as the atmosphere they live in every day.

- Live your life together in the spirit of love and romance. Recapture the magic that brought you together in the first place. Set the romantic mood for each "loving" event as well.

- Romance and passion may produce feelings of love, but partnership is what makes love work.

- Arousal can be achieved in many different ways. It's up to the partners to decide how. Both partners need to be aroused to have a good experience.

- Use touching to learn about each other's anatomy.

- Avoid "turnoffs"—follow some commonsense suggestions.

- Sensual touching is extremely arousing for most couples.

- Play to your partner's dominant sense (sight, sound, or touch) to heighten his or her enjoyment.

- Loving entails giving and receiving, and handling differenc

Chapter 4
Regaining Intimacy

N ow that you understand a little better some of the basic physiology and psychology of arousal, and the reality of aging and prostate cancer treatment, it's time to look at how you can move forward with a fulfilling sex life. In this chapter, we'll talk about two different methods for enhancing sex, which can be combined for a great loving experience: 1) relearning loving, and 2) home remedies. Commercial therapies and medications will be discussed in Chapter 5.

Relearning Loving

The reality is that older men generally no longer get aroused at the mere thought of a woman in their arms or at the sight of one that would have "turned them on" in the past.

Even before therapy, most of us had become used to our partner, to the things we did when we made love, and to the environment-doing it in the same place and at the same time. On the one hand, such familiarity can make for wonderful loving because you know each other's likes and dislikes. On the other hand, too much repetition of same-style lovemaking can lead to boredom. When sex becomes a routine event, partners may become less interested. This decreasing interest may coincide with the changes we experience with aging.

Let's admit it: many of us had a lukewarm love life even before prostate cancer treatment. So how do you rekindle the fire-or, if you have it, how do you make sure it does not go out?

Earlier we said that knowing your partner could make loving better rather than worse. The key is that it should be easier to talk about loving, and your likes and dislikes, with a person you are comfortable with.

One woman told us that the security of the relationship lets her "do things with her body" that she would not dare do with a new partner. She said she feels "free to explore new ideas." Prostate cancer therapy forced this couple to rethink how they made love and to share their thoughts.

Start with the idea that when suddenly faced with impotence, you have to *relearn how to make love. The best place to start is by learning what your partner likes.* In the course of talking in support groups, as well as in private conversations, men have commented that they "don't know how to begin." When they were younger, erections came easily; the erection seemed to be the "switch." After some kissing and playing, the "switch" turned on, and they would go directly to intercourse. This may have taken just a few minutes.

Now, they find that this method is no longer enough to give them an erection. So "what do we do?" This lack of knowing what to do reflects the fact that many couples have forgotten "how to make love."

Making love is an art. It is like painting. The painter uses brushes and paints to create an effect on a canvas. He or she has to know what will happen when a certain brush is used. The painter decides on the effect he or she wants to create and selects the right brush. The brush is the means by which the painter creates the effect with one or more paints. One may think of the "loving" brushes as the kiss and different kinds of touch. For example, a kiss on the neck may produce one effect. Running the tongue from the lips down the throat to the breast will produce a different sensation.

The other variable in all of this is the partner. One approach to loving does not work for all men or all women. Each of us reacts to different stimuli, humor, certain touches, etc. Each one should know, and ask, what the partner likes and doesn't like. Understanding what action

When suddenly faced with impotence, you have to relearn how to make love and find out what your partner likes.

Making love is an art—and you are the artists.

Relearning loving is regaining passion and rediscovering secrets to arousal.

The longer you don't make love, the less likely you are to start again.

will produce what effect in the partner is one of the key benefits of long-term relationships.

Sometimes preferences and sensitivities change over time. It's important to keep asking each other what "feels best."

Most aids and medications that produce or enlarge erections will only work when the man is aroused or stimulated. As the manufacturer of Viagra says, Viagra does not create desire-it only helps with the performance. The essence of relearning loving is regaining passion and rediscovering secrets to arousal.

As the expression goes, "when you're hot, you're hot, and when you're not, you're not." When you're not, many medications will not work at all, and others will not work as well. So before you resort to medication you may not need, you should learn how to get stimulated and passionate. That's what this chapter is all about.

Let's assume you have a situation where the frequency of having sex has declined over a number of years for many reasons. In addition, you have refrained from sex since your therapy because of failure to perform. This leads to disappointment, embarrassment, and frustration. These concerns, coupled with a low frequency of having sex before therapy, make it doubly difficult to recover the capability and the pleasure.

Your partner, anxious not to upset you, retreats. She feels it is better not to push, hoping that in time, you will begin to address the problem. Unfortunately, this is a self-defeating approach. The longer you don't make love, the easier it is to continue not loving and the more difficult it is to resume loving.

The first action is to reset yourself mentally. This begins with exploring what each of you enjoys when you make love.

One way to get started is to share what each one enjoyed in the past. This could reawaken the pathway for getting excited. Then it's a really good idea to have a "touch session" where you explore each other's bodies and tell each other where the most sensitive points are.

Many men find that after prostate cancer treatment, sensitivity may be heightened in new areas. Your partner will never know unless you tell her. If you don't know, take the time to touch each other and explore. You must begin slowly, perhaps only kissing and touching the first few times. During this time, you should tell each other what you like.

Don't focus on the erection. Instead, focus on loving and deriving pleasure from it. When erections were easy, we tended to focus solely on them. In reality, most of us missed out on other means of deriving pleasure, which could have made loving much more pleasurable even then.

A screenwriter in his mid-50s, quoted in an article in *New Choices,* expressed it very well: "Passion-sexual passion-is about emotion. Really knowing how to make love to a woman allows you to stop thinking and become more deeply passionate. . . . it's all about feeling and letting yourself go."

At the same time, since loving is a two-person activity, you also have part of the assignment for getting your partner aroused and wanting to share and participate in the experience with you. So go ahead-have a "touch session"-pretend that you've never made love before and are first learning about each other's bodies.

An erection may happen as a "side effect" of getting aroused-but usually not if you're anxious about it.

Couples should shift their focus from the erection to giving and receiving pleasure.

Loving is a Partnering Activity, Not a Solo Sport

You need a partner to make love. Yet, as obvious as it sounds, many men of our generation feel they are driving the loving session; communication is not what they focus on. But the bridge for working with, being with, loving someone is communication. Without it, you might as well try to make love to yourself.

Communication may be initially difficult because men who experience erectile dysfunction are often depressed and generally find it difficult to talk about their inability to "perform." Men do not generally admit they have

Good long-term sex is . . . about eroticism.

There are many ways to please a woman, and most of them have absolutely nothing to do with erections.

erectile dysfunction. By the time they admit it, they have gone through a lot of emotional upset.

Psychologists say that many spouses are reluctant to talk to their partners about what pleases them because they are " too vulnerable to rejection, too concerned that they'll cause discomfort in their partner and/or incur disapproval. For . . . any of us-daring to reveal what we want sexually is to risk losing a relationship with that partner." They also say that "Good long-term sex is not about manual dexterity but about eroticism.
And . . . eroticism is about revealing yourself and what turns you on-it requires a couple to be vulnerable." (Self Jan 1998, p.112). And to let yourself be vulnerable, partners must feel confident and comfortable with each other.

Men and women have equal responsibility to make loving work. People born before the 50s often look to the man to take total responsibility for the act and for the enjoyment of the woman. The culture of those born in the 50s, 60s, and later is much more in tune with the idea of sharing the responsibility (and the pleasure). But older couples often have to learn it deliberately.

In a prostate cancer support group, a man shared the pain impotence caused him. He said, "I want so much to please my wife, and now I can't. It is so frustrating!" Barbara asked him if he had asked his wife what would please her. He had not, because he assumed that an erection was the only way to satisfy her. There are so many ways to give pleasure to a woman, and most of them have absolutely nothing to do with erections.

Sexual touching brings great pleasure to most women. To enable women to reach orgasm, couples are successfully using oral sex, stimulation of the clitoris with the finger or hand, vibrators, and even-surprise!-completely limp penises!

This last point is not immediately obvious to many couples, so we'll get a bit more technical here. You can touch the tip or the side of the penis against the clitoris, producing very pleasurable sensations for both partners. The woman needs to be well lubricated, either with her own natural vaginal fluid or saliva, or with a commercial lubricant like Astroglide or KY Jelly.

In the beginning, you may want the woman to control the movement, but as you learn together, by all means take turns. You can also experiment with different positions-for instance, the man sitting on a chair or the woman on top of the man, or the man standing behind the woman. Gravity helps the woman to stay lubricated, so if you are in a position where the man is "on top," be prepared to lubricate more frequently.

One of the great things about relearning loving is that you get to try new things and experiment together. If you talk to each other about it, and are open to the new experiences this will bring you as a couple, you will find that this sharing enriches your relationship tremendously. The communication will extend to other areas of your life and generally get you better "in tune" with each other.

This enables you to be more sensitive and to choose the most appropriate approach to your partner at any given time. The ingredients for stimulation depend on our psychological state of being at a given moment and what else is going on in our lives. A person who just got a big raise or the job they wanted needs a different approach than one who may need comfort and support because of a personal downturn. In each instance, the incentives for physical activity will be different. Passionate loving in one instance may be replaced by the need for hugging and cuddling in another.

Touching

What is the largest sexual part of the body? It's the skin. Being touched is a primal experience. Believe it or not, one hormone has been identified as the "touch hormone" and is sometimes called the "cuddle chemical." In *The Art of Staying Together,* Diane Ackerman writes about mothers secreting the chemical in response to a baby's cries that makes the "mother want to nuzzle and hug it. . . . Oxytocin seems to play an equally important role in romantic love, as a hormone that encourages cuddling between lovers and increases pleasure during

The body's largest sexual organ is the skin. Touching is a primal experience.

41

Oxytocin is the key chemical in long-lasting love. The body craves the touch of one particular person.

lovemaking. The hormone . . . snowballs during sexual arousal-the more intense the arousal, the more oxytocin is produced. As arousal builds, oxytocin is thought to cause . . . orgasm."

The chemical's involvement in arousal is unique because it is "generated both by physical and emotional cues-a certain look, voice, or gesture is enough and can become conditioned to one's personal love history. . . . The lover's smell or touch may trigger the production of oxytocin. So might a . . . sexual fantasy. " Women secrete more of this chemical and are more responsive to it than men, which explains why "women more than men prefer to continue embracing after sex."

From the foregoing, psychologists contend that oxytocin is the key chemical in long-lasting love. The body craves touch and quickly learns to crave the touch of one particular person. It's addictive.

Pleasurable touching between a woman and a man is always possible, regardless of the effects of cancer treatment. Touching is not time-restricted nor time-constrained. It can be done any time, any place, for a second, a minute or more. A touch on the hand or arm. A brief touch on the shoulders. It provides connectedness. It is on the path to the more intimate moments.

Dr. Ruth Westheimer writes that "Kissing is so erotic because of the many nerve endings in the lips. Typically, women like kissing more than men, but there's no physiological reason for this. Many men simply feel pressured to rush into sex because they have an erection. Instead, if you both get used to slowing down, you'll enjoy kissing more." (*New Woman*, June 1994).

As mentioned in the "What's Your Style" section of Chapter 3, we respond differently to certain stimuli. For example, there are the "looking" types and there are the "feeling/touching" types. If the mere sight of your lover, or of certain parts of his or her anatomy, inspires you, you're a watcher. The feeler/toucher gets excited when the partner massages him or her, when they hold hands, or when they feel something like satin sheets or lingerie.

Carrying the touching a bit further, take a shower together and soap each other. Run your hand over your partner's skin and enjoy the way it feels. Use the opportunity to find areas that each of you like to have touched.

You could even consider making showering part of the loving once in awhile. One couple takes it a step further by putting skin lotion on the one who has just showered. They do this as part of their everyday relationship. It doesn't usually lead to sex right then, but it sends the message that they enjoy touching each other.

As mentioned elsewhere, one objective of intimate touching is to help you find out the parts of your anatomy that are sensitive, that give you pleasure. You can find out about the way you respond to stimulation and let your partner know.

Make showering together part of your loving once in a while.

Be Creative in Your Love Life

Being creative is extremely important for several reasons. Creativity leads to newness and something different, which in turn produces interest, desire, attraction, and stimulation. Creativity can make up for a lot of difficulties and make a relationship exciting. It transforms the routine lovemaking and leads to more desire and easier arousal. Creativity leads to "freshness," keeping the relationship interesting and lively.

Many couples get to the point of treating the sex part of loving as something they must do. Such a "chore" becomes dull and boring, as any job would. Many people try to change the structure of their work, whether at home or at the office, to keep from being bored. Why not use the same approach where loving is concerned? It's up to you to make it new, to freshen it up. If sex has become boring, now is your chance to start fresh and liven it up by turning sex into loving.

Peter and Julia, who decided to change their loving style in their 60s, told us they talk often now about how great and new it feels, and one would not know they have been together for so many years. Once when the kids were visiting, he pulled her behind the kitchen door and kissed her passionately. They liked it so well that now they play this game of "hiding" even when nobody is

Vary the time and place for making love.

We dress for playing tennis, swimming, and going to the theater. How about dressing up for loving?

around. Barbara often collects a "toll" kiss when Ralph passes by. It's all part of creating an environment of "permanent romance."

How can you get out of the rut? If you are mentally locked into a time and place for loving, maybe it's time to think about a change to spice it up.

Often we reserve loving activities for the bedroom and after dark. How about taking time in the afternoon? Many couples find that sex is more enjoyable during the day because both are wide awake and have more energy. Studies have proven that as we get older, our body clock shifts backward. This means that we are likely to get tired much earlier and be ready to go to bed about 10 p.m. or even earlier. Similarly, we are inclined to get up earlier. Loving and sex require energy. Doing it late at night, when you are likely to be most tired, means that you are not able to focus on what you are doing. It is harder to get aroused. And certainly, you are less able to perform.

How about playing around in the kitchen while the two of you are making dinner? Or on the couch while watching TV or a video? Or how about going to a hotel overnight? The important thing is to get out of the rut where it is done in the same place at the same time in the same way.

Why not dress up for loving? We dress for playing tennis, swimming, and going to the theater. Presenting oneself as attractively as possible is a basic factor in mating. Humankind does it by dressing and grooming. We did it while we dated. What's wrong with doing it now? Looking good also gives us more confidence in the bedroom as well as outside it.

It is okay to make love with things that stimulate you. There have probably always been clothes your partner wore that turned you on. If there's something special that you like, go out and buy it. Putting on a garter belt and stiletto heels may not be your cup of tea, but it's your responsibility to figure out what your cup of tea is and tell it (or show it) to your partner.

The idea is that you can start a loving session differently than you usually do.

There is also the environmental aspect: creating the romance. Use flowers, candles, music, and wine (only a little-too much is not good). Maybe there's a perfume you like and that will appeal to your partner. Many people get excited by certain scents and smells.

In general, it is okay to think of loving as something that you are going to do and prepare for. Thinking about it is one way of getting the juices flowing. When we were younger, guys would say, "I can't wait until I get my hands on her." They were daydreaming and imagining how great it would be. By the time the date happened, they could barely contain themselves. You can re-create this feeling with your partner if you let your creativity flow.

Part of the romance is also what you do *after* the loving. Women of all ages complain that after lovemaking, their men just roll over and go to sleep. They would like the cuddling and holding to go on for a while.

Remember how it was when you were young lovers-or how it should have been! Lying completely relaxed after loving, talking about your relationship, or the love you just made, where you got pleasure, or your dreams of the next time. . . . You can re-create that feeling now, talking after loving. It's not a great idea to talk about money, the kids, or mundane everyday things! This is your precious time together for sharing and intimate conversation, as if there were nothing else in the world.

Remember the "cuddle chemical" and how it stimulates women? Combine the cuddling after loving with a sweet appeal to her ears. Whisper in her ear how great it was, and how much you love her. She will store those words away, and the next time you're in a romantic mood, repeat a few of those words, and it will trigger all these sweet memories and she'll just melt in your arms. The women should do their share of whispering, too!

As you may know, some commercial medications require the man to take them in advance, and suggest that you should not get "stimulated" too soon, But there's nothing wrong with setting the right mood. It is also okay to prepare for loving without medication and much better for your focus on real lovemaking. It's a good idea

Recapture the spirit of your younger years—when loving and intimacy were fun.

Good loving takes time. Deadlines are deadly.

not to take medication every time. This way, the erection becomes a special event and introduces variety into love-making.

If you're still finding it hard to get out of the "rut" and recharge your lovelife by yourself, don't give up. It's okay to see a sex therapist. They can work with you based on your specific situation. If you don't "click" with the first therapist, try another. If this area of your life is important to you, it's worth an investment of time and a little money.

Take Time

We need time to make good love. Time pressure is an enemy. When we were younger and erections could be willed (and sometimes were involuntary), intercourse could be said to be possible at the drop of a hat. You will find that trying to get excited under pressure almost assures that you will not get aroused, or that you will have a lot of difficulty doing so. Anxiety will hang over you. The more you worry about doing it in a certain amount of time, the more difficult it will be. So you do need the luxury of setting aside the time, then forgetting about time altogether. To enjoy making love, allow yourselves enough time to savor its pleasures.

Even if touch is not your partner's primary means of arousal, you can use touch to get there. In recent years, therapists have recommended touching and massage as a means for couples to begin intimacy and physical reconnection. Masters & Johnson say it well: "for the man and woman who value each other as individuals and who want the satisfactions of a sustained relationship . . . *Touch is an end in itself.* . . . Touching is sensual pleasure, exploring the texture of skin. . . ." They continue: "And yet such is the nature of the sense of touch, which can simultaneously give and receive impressions, that the very pleasure a woman may experience in stroking her husband's face, for example, is relayed back through her fingertips to give him the pleasure of being aware of her pleasure in him. . . . [I]n touching and being touched by a trusted and trusting person of the opposite sex, one experiences not only the pleasure of being alive but the joy of being a sexual creature. . . ." (*The Pleasure Bond,* p. 238-240).

Just Do it: Make Love

The key point of relearning loving is to do it whenever and wherever you can. Whenever you practice a new skill or technique in life or relearn something you used to do, you have to practice. It's true for lovemaking, too. Not everything you try will work. Don't worry about it; maybe share a good laugh about something that didn't work-and then try something else. Practice makes perfect!

Making love is personal and individual. No two couples do it exactly the same. No two couples get exactly the same feelings from it, even if they do it approximately the same way. Everyone's physical responses are different. Just as all artists have to practice with different brushes and mixing colors and how to apply them to get the desired result, if we want to improve our lovemaking, we have to do the same.

However you want to practice it, doing it-making love-enables partners to be connected. Equally important, it counters atrophy of the penis. Make love as often as you both feel like it. Don't be afraid to damage anything. If anything hurts, just stop that particular activity.

Good lovemaking takes practice—just like all skills.

Make love as often as you both feel like it.

Home Remedies

What we mean by home remedies are the things that you can do at home with no or minimal cost. These include exercises for toning the lovemaking muscles, relaxation techniques to reduce anxiety, and some herbs that may help, and some common-sense practices.

Kegel Exercises

Gynecologists have long recommended Kegel exercises to women to improve pelvic muscular control and give them and their partners greater sexual pleasure. They are named after Dr. Arnold H. Kegel, an American gynecologist.

Urologists recommend that men do Kegel exercises after a radical prostatectomy.

We've heard the exercises described in a number of ways. Physical rehabilitation professionals recommend the following formula for doing the Kegel exercises.

1. Tighten the muscles as if you wanted to stop the flow during urination. (These are the pubococcygeal muscles.)

2. Hold these muscles tight for a count of 10.

3. Then, while continuing to hold the above position, tighten the anal/rectal muscles. Hold both sets of muscles tight for an additional count of 10.

4. Do 10 repetitions at least three times daily.

In addition, generally toning your body will improve your lovemaking capability. Include exercises for your abdominal muscles, for your upper arm (triceps and biceps), and for your back. Back exercises, which usually include abdominal routines, also include back extensions and push-ups.

Use Gravity

When you want to produce and maintain an erection, use body positions that will help blood flow to the penis. This could mean making love on your knees or in the "missionary position" (man on top), or even standing up. The latter can be done with the man standing at the side of the bed and the woman kneeling or lying on the bed. Usually, American bed height is sufficient for this type of intercourse.

A man will retain an erection much longer in the standing, kneeling, or missionary position.

In the standing, kneeling, or missionary position, a man will retain an erection much longer than otherwise. Certainly, a man with erectile problems will not have as firm an erection when he is lying down.

Even with MUSE, gravity helps: it is recommended that the man walk around or at least stand or sit, rather than lie down, while waiting for the medication to take effect. (See Chapter 5 for a detailed description of MUSE.)

But again, don't get hung up about the erection. Other positions offer many other wonderful ways to interact, so don't restrict yourself to only those positions that increase the blood flow to the penis.

Massage the Penis

A penis needs normal blood flow to stay alive. Nature provides for this through nocturnal erections, normally three to five times per night, which oxygenate the penis. If the penis does not get enough oxygen, collagen builds up, and the resultant scarring damages the spongy tissue, the penis loses elasticity, and normal blood flow is impossible.

If therapy has damaged blood flow to the penis, the man must rely on manual stimulation to retain erectile capability. This will stimulate the blood flow, prevent atrophy, and thereby improve erectile capability.

Massage the penis frequently. Many people, remembering admonitions from their childhood, ask "Is it really okay to do this?". The answer is, not only is it OK, it's recommended. This is truly a "use it or lose it" situation. Recently, urologists have begun recommending that their surgery patients use manual stimulation as soon as the catheter has been removed, several times daily if possible. This helps to normalize blood flow into the penis, which helps keep the muscle alive.

Massaging the penis stimulates the bloodflow, which increases the chance to recover potency.

Partial Penetration

Many men can have some degree of erection, which allows for partial penetration. (The only name we have ever heard for this technique, "stuffing," does not sound terribly romantic.)

Even when you don't have a full erection but there is some engorgement of the penis, it is probably "stuffable" or "mashable." Since the woman's clitoris is on the outside, women can get significant pleasure without much penetration.

Successful loving after prostate cancer therapy requires both partners to be active.

Saying that you're not that interested in sex won't help him much.

The Partner's Role

Successful loving after prostate cancer therapy requires both partners to be active. The partner plays a key role in rebuilding the man's confidence. Remaining sexually active is also necessary for a woman's welfare. The Mayo Clinic notes that "Regular sexual activity improves vaginal lubrication and elasticity after estrogen declines."

There are a number of key events in which the partner's reaction makes a critical difference to the future of the relationship. The woman's reaction may cause the man to either withdraw or to be encouraged. Sending a positive message can make a big difference in reestablishing the man's ego, and in rebuilding the sexual foundation for the couple. Being supportive and loving is critical in these situations.

After a man has treatment, the partner should participate actively, show her desire by initiating sexual touching and lovemaking, and express her interest and support. By all means say that you are interested in lovemaking, whether there is an erection or not. Saying that you're not that interested in sex won't help him much (unless it's the truth, and even then you should discuss how and how often you still want to do something). Telling him that you want to find ways to please him, and sharing how he can please you, is also a good starting point. Reassuring him that he is still able to please you can make a big difference in the way he feels about himself.

- If there is no erection, tell him that an erection is not the most important thing to you. Show him what to do so your needs are met. This can mean bringing you to orgasm, or touching and holding you in a certain way-whatever it is you need to feel happy and satisfied. You can also suggest that you bring him to orgasm if he would like.

- He can learn from you that it's not always necessary to have an orgasm to be satisfied. Encourage him to try it. Most men associate "orgasm-less" sex with frustration. They will be in for a pleasant surprise if they let go of this goal orientation.

- If you are using any aids that are supposed to produce an erection, you must both be aware that they might or might not work. You're going to try it a few times, but if it does not work, you realize that it is not his "fault." Please don't ever, ever use sex as a weapon. It's destructive to your relationship.

- Your reaction to his suggestion to make love is very important in the beginning. So what do you do when you're not up for it? Be honest, but tell him it's not general lack of interest-just that you are very tired, or not feeling well, or whatever the real reason is-but that you really love to make love to him. Ask him for a rain-check for tomorrow or the weekend. Then you can reaffirm your interest by initiating loving the next day or weekend.

- Equally important is your reaction should he experience any incontinence during loving. More about these "leaks" later.

So you've tried to be the perfect supportive partner. But let's face it, you're human, and you slipped up. Your reaction got him upset. An apology is never too late. At the first opportunity, as soon as you realize that you did not say the right thing, you should correct the situation. Here is what happened to Judy and how she handled it. Judy and Joe hadn't made love for five months, since before his prostate cancer surgery. Finally one night he got up the nerve to start playing around, but found soon that nothing happened "down there." Judy realized that he was very upset about it, and out of a sense of protection told him that it was all right, that she didn't care that much about sex anyway. They both rolled over and pretended to go to sleep.

Aids that are supposed to produce an erection may or may not work.

But Judy was kicking herself! She loved Joe very much and really wanted to have a physical relationship; she just didn't want to hurt him with "demands." After talking it over with her friend Lisa, who happened to be a therapist, she figured out a way to start a conversation with Joe. It went something like this: "Honey, when we started to make love a few days ago, and you couldn't get an erection, I told you I didn't care much for sex any more. But that's not true at all. I just said it because I saw you were getting so upset, and I wanted you to stop hurting. Instead I think I hurt you more. What I should have told you is how I really feel: I want us to continue showing each other our love through lovemaking. We don't have to do it the same way we used to. If you don't have an erection, that's not the end of it. We'll find other ways to please each other.

It's so important to me that we keep that connection. Can you forgive me for what I said? Are you willing to work with me on this?"

You bet he was-and he was so glad that she hadn't meant what she said that night!

Such a conversation can open the door again. The two words "I'm sorry" are very powerful! There are many times the man has reason to apologize, too-for example, if he was expecting an erection and it did not happen, and he found a way to blame his partner. For some reason, it seems much harder to extract the two little words from a man than from a woman. What is it, guys, something genetic? If you mess up, please do fess up-we find you irresistible when you say you're sorry!

Now let's talk about the "big secret" that nobody wants to talk about: leaks.

Leaks occur because surgery patients lose one of their sphincters during the operation. After surgery, many men experience small leaks-involuntary release of urine-during lovemaking, even if they have total bladder control during daily activities. A Johns Hopkins Hospital surgeon estimates that over the long term, about 95 percent of men will have total bladder control, especially during the day. But right after surgery, many men have urine-control problems. It's quite similar to stress incontinence,

The two words "I'm sorry" are very powerful!

Many surgery patients have urinary leaks during sexual activity, even if they normally have nearly total urinary control.

which many women have. Many women are used to leaks, but men often get embarrassed and withdraw. Ladies, don't let a little thing like that shut down your love life! Support, and if your partner can accept it, a little dose of humor, will get both of you through the first few occurrences.

There are some commonsense things you should do to minimize this type of interruption:

- Obviously, both men and women should make sure they are clean.

- If you have a tendency to leak, it's a good idea to void before you make love. Some men have found that if they sit on the commode, they will void more completely. Otherwise, they may find themselves leaking and be prompted to void a second and possibly a third time. Also, as mentioned earlier, keep tissues or a small towel nearby.

Void before you make love.

- One man told us that cranberries or cranberry juice taken every day may help reduce or control stress leaks. A study affirmed the folk tale that cranberries have a beneficial effect on the urinary tract. Ideally, take extract pills or dried cranberries, or drink 100 percent cranberry juice, which is so tart that you will have to cut it with another juice or even some sugar.

Try cranberries or cranberry juice to reduce leaks.

Another approach to coping with leaks is to use a nasal decongestant before loving. Studies have found that it helps women with mild stress incontinence. The likelihood is that it can help men since it restricts urination. For the same reason men with urinary difficulty, such as happens with enlarged prostates, should not use it.

If either partner has a serious problem with incontinence, a number of things can be done. You should consult your doctor.

Fatty foods and red meats create fatty deposits in the penis that clog the blood vessels that help create an erection. You decide what you want: steak or sex.

Eating Right

Fatty foods and red meats create fatty deposits in the penis that clog the blood vessels that help create an erection. You decide what you want: steak or sex. Seriously, it's a good idea to cut down on meat and fats for many reasons, including potency.

If you are intending to make love, it's a good idea not to eat a heavy meal, especially not one with lots of meat and potatoes. Most people are sluggish after eating such a meal. Most of the blood rushes to the stomach to help digest the food instead of going to the brain to help get you aroused, and to the penis.

We have also talked about drinking alcohol before loving. The more alcohol you drink, the less likely the loving will be good, and the less likely it will happen.

Herbal Products

Some herbal products are reputed to, and *may* actually, help loving. This section discusses three natural products that are often mentioned in this regard.

Our comments are not meant to be comprehensive. Literature and anecdotes abound concerning products that are libido lifters, will give you King Kong-type erections, and will drive your partner wild with excitement. We don't know anything about these products and suspect that most of the related information is marketing hype.

We will tell you about some products that have been discussed in the prostate cancer literature. We are not recommending that you take any product. While herbal products are natural, they are not always harmless. They may worsen a current condition, have bad side effects, or interfere with medications you are taking. For example, patients with high blood pressure should not take ginseng.

In general, if you use herbal products, you should buy the standardized extract of the herb made by a reputable company. Several studies have reported that some companies' labels were misleading. Products made by reputable companies' will be reliably labeled.

Readers interested in more information on herbs and supplements should consult *The American Pharmaceutical Association Practical Guide to Natural Medicines* by Andrea Peirce, which covers more than 300 herbs and some supplements. The book provides the scientific and common names for each herb, the ailment(s) it's recommended for, the forms in which it is available, the commonly prescribed dosages, and information on the herb's effectiveness and safety based on scientific study.

Erogenex

Erogenex is a new herbal product introduced by Erogen in December 1998.

Each capsule contains extracts of 300 mg of *avena sativa* and 150 mg of *sabal serrulata*. (*Avena sativa* is a form of wild oats and *sabal serrulata* is a derivative of the Florida palm tree known as saw palmetto or sabal (*serenoa repens*)).

According to the manufacturer, Erogenex works to increase sexual desire by "increasing the bioavailable testosterone." The company claims "the pill boosts libido, endurance, stamina; increases lubrication in women; and aids men in achieving and maintaining erections" and "has been found to be effective in 70 percent of men."

Currently, the product, also known as Ex22, is "only available directly through the company." The company offers a 30-day guarantee. The company's recommended dosage is two capsules daily. One month's supply costs $39.95.

None of our sources was aware of any studies supporting the company's claim that the active ingredients help to stimulate sexual desire as well as enhance performance. We were also not able to obtain any information on possible side effects. The company claims the product is safe.

This product has not gone through clinical trials. However, because medical claims have been made, the product has been referred to the food division of the Food and Drug Administration (FDA) for review. As of this writing, the FDA has not commented.

For more information: Tel: 888-636-2229

Gingko

Studies have shown that gingko may have therapeutic effects. Gingkolide B was isolated by Harvard scientists in the 1980s. Gingko's effect is to dramatically increase blood flow to the brain, and it is purportedly able to improve "blood flow through peripheral arteries lined with plaque."

One 1998 article stated that because it increases blood flow and circulation, gingko may work in a way similar to Viagra. *Psychology Today* in its October 1998 issue reported: "In one recent study, 50 patients with impotence were given gingko, and after six months, an astonishing one-half had regained sexual vigor. . . . [M]en taking gingko need to be patient, since significant results may not show up for several months. It takes time for the body to repair damaged blood vessels. . . ." Anecdotal confirmation comes from several people who responded to our article in the January-February 1998 issue of the Education Center for Prostate Cancer Patients (ECPCP) newsletter, saying that doubling the normal dose of gingko (from 60 to 120 mg twice a day) enabled them to obtain erections. Ginko is manufactured by many herbal product companies and is widely available, including even in supermarkets.

Kava

The kava plant has been widely reported to be a natural relaxant that does not dull the mind, as many such substances do. As a result, kava permits an individual's natural sexual appetite to surface.

One of the biggest problems for both prostate cancer survivors and others is that psychological factors as well as physical factors, limit a man's capability for intercourse. Fifteen chemicals in the kava plant are said to ease anxiety and relax muscles. Erections occur when the penile muscles relax. Concurrently, erections are facilitated when the psychological barrier is lessened, because there is less anxiety about getting an erection.

Staying In Shape

Numerous studies have shown that physically active people are more receptive to sex, have greater sexual desire, and most important, are better able to participate in sexual activity. A 1998 technical paper dealing with prostate cancer patients' quality of life showed that "sexual function correlated positively with physical vigor . . . implying that impotence may have an effect on general HRQOL (health-related quality of life)."

Although we do not think of it as such, sexual activity is physically demanding. Heart rate and breathing increase as with any physical exertion. With the availability of erectile dysfunction medication, men who have not been engaging in sex and who are not getting any exercise are suddenly becoming sexually active. Unfortunately, they are poorly prepared for the physical demands of such activity which can result in a heart attack or stroke.

If you are interested in improving your love life, you should maintain a regular exercise program. The type of activity you engage in is less important than that you do something. Walking, using free weights (three- and five-pounders, or cans of vegetables), and sit-ups (also called crunches and good for toning the gut) are all recommended. Washing and waxing a car or washing floors for 45-60 minutes are examples of exercise mentioned in the July 1996 Surgeon General's report on physical activity.

If you go to a local gym or a senior or community center, that's great. Participating in a regular aerobics, yoga, or other exercise class will help tone your muscles and increase your physical stamina and endurance. As is noted in many exercise publications, if you have been physically inactive, get medical guidance before you begin any exercise program.

Cardiovascular research has proven that exercise can reduce stress and anxiety, lower blood pressure, and lessen cholesterol, all of which means better lovemaking. High blood pressure (hypertension) has been associated with erectile dysfunction.

The benefits of exercising are many and include a sense of well-being, not unlike the runner's high. This

Physical activity can improve sexual function.

comes in large part from the endorphins that are generated during a workout. Another benefit is the sense of feeling better about yourself. In part, this is because you will look better. One man who divorced in middle age found that his diet and exercise program had given him a body that looked twenty years younger and this enabled him to survive his second tour of singledom. It also contributed significantly to satisfaction in his relationships. He felt good about himself, and his partners were equally interested.

An interesting by-product of endorphins is that they also increase the sexual desire. This is tied in with an increase in energy, feeling better in general, and feeling better about yourself and the way you look. Add to this the additional stamina, physical flexibility, and capacity to engage in sex. If it sounds like you are preparing for your personal lovemaking Olympics, you are.

Regaining Intimacy

Key Points

- Loving is an art.
- Relearning how to make love means taking time for talking, touching, loving. Do it when there are no pressures.
- Focusing on the erection takes away from the pleasure of intimacy.
- Going to a sex therapist may be a good idea, and it does not have to be a long-term program.
- Do Kegel exercises.
- Make it easier to get an erection by using positions in lovemaking which take advantage of gravity, thus helping blood flow into the penis.
- Massage the penis to avoid atrophy.
- If you have partial erections, try partial penetration.
- The partner plays a key role in bringing the man back to successful lovemaking after prostate cancer.
- Avoid fatty foods, which will clog the arteries in the penis and the rest of the body.
- Some herbal over-the-counter products are low-risk.
- Staying in shape improves your physical life, including the sexual part.

Chapter 5
Commercial
Therapies and
Medications

In addition to the things you can do for yourself to create the best possible physical, physiological, and mental environment for loving, it's also important to discuss commercial therapies and medications for erectile dysfunction.

These therapies cover the spectrum from mechanical support devices to injections to pills. A broad variety of therapies and mixtures exist, and pharmaceutical companies periodically introduce new ones. In this chapter we cover the major commercial means that can aid men in obtaining erections. Certainly, if you know of others that should be included in later editions of this book, please let us know.

Ideally, it would be nice to have one therapy for erectile failure. One article notes five characteristics required for universal treatment. The treatment should be:

- Effective

- Useful immediately when needed

- Free of toxicity and side effects

- Easy to use in the form of pills or cream

- Affordable

Unfortunately, this ideal therapy does not exist. What is available may be effective only some of the time and for some men. Most medications and therapies work soon after being taken (they increase performance soon after being used, within 10 minutes to one hour). Some of the companies are working on oral medications that will shrink the waiting time. Although some are easy to use, all of them have side effects.

Where money is concerned, it's important to separate initial cost versus per-use cost. For example, a pump may cost up to $500 initially, but nothing thereafter, whereas a Viagra pill costs $8 to $9 each.

We've organized this chapter according to the approaches for improving the ability to obtain and maintain erections:

- oral medications/treatments

- topical medications: penile creams and gels

- Devices

  penile splints and supports

  vacuum pumps

- intraurethral medication

- penile injection

- penile implants

- penile vascular surgery

A 1996 article by Dr. Jonathan P. Jarow assessed patient preference, satisfaction, and overall outcome of therapy. This study is significant because many past assessments were based on the doctor's perception. As you can imagine, oral medication was the overall favorite, being initially preferred 79 percent of the time, but only 16 percent had satisfactory results. The oral medications used at the time were yohimbine and trazodone. The other treatments-constrictive bands, self-injection therapy, vacuum devices, and surgery-were initially chosen by less than five percent each. Satisfaction with the selected therapy in these small groups ranged from

37 percent for the constrictive bands to 100 percent for surgery. Eight percent elected not to have any therapy at all.

After a two-year follow-up, at the conclusion of the study, only 40 percent of the patients were satisfied with their sexual function. Most of the 60 percent who were not satisfied "chose to avoid more effective therapies even if available."

The incredible demand for Viagra confirms the findings of this earlier study that oral medications are vastly preferred, even if other medications are available and more appropriate for some men.

Viagra is not the be-all and end-all; other therapies are slated to come to market within the first couple of years of the new century.

With most therapies and medications, you must be sexually aroused. In fact, the effectiveness of treatment is somewhat proportional to your level of excitement. Other than by using injections or implants, you cannot have instantaneous erections without first getting excited.

A medication or aid that works for one person will not always work for someone else.

The initial use of a medication may not have the expected results, either initially, after a few times, or at all. Since a medication works only on a certain percentage of men in clinical trials, it cannot be expected to work on all the men who will use it after it becomes available. In other words, don't start doubting yourself if something does not work because there is no one miracle aid that works for everybody. Try it a few times, see if there is an effect, ask the doctor to adjust the dosage, and if it still doesn't work, ask the doctor to prescribe something else.

Because applicability, suitability, and effectiveness vary for different people, some doctors prescribe "cocktails" for patients. For example, one doctor prescribes an injection for one person, but an injected medication and a pill for someone else. Only a doctor who knows your medical history can counsel you effectively. You, your doctor, and your partner jointly should make any decision about what is best for you.

A medication or aid that works for one person will not always work for someone else.

With aids that are generally referred to as "performance medication," many men have newfound capability. Therefore, they must think about the consequences of using these products. If a medication does work, one consequence is that there may be more demands on one or both partners in the relationship. For example, in a situation where the relationship has settled down to minimal or no sex, how will the partners react to changing the balance? If the medication works, will one or both of the partners be happy and excited about the renewed capability, or afraid of the new sexual relationship?

Some partners may be afraid or at least not enthused about returning to physical aspects of the early relationship if they have been living in a relationship where sex has been absent. We have been told about women asking their husband's doctor to stop prescribing erectile aids. The decision to use a certain medication, and to continue using it, should be made by both partners.

You need to realize that when you had to face the fact that you had lost some or all of your erectile capability, you were affected psychologically. Now that you start thinking of being able to have erections again, you may feel good. On the other hand, you may feel uncertain, and even anxious. You may even feel threatened because you are uncertain how your partner will react. Equally, your partner may feel threatened and start worrying about new demands being imposed.

Assuming you and your partner agree that you should use a commercial impotence therapy, realistic expectations should be the order of the day. The therapy may not work, may work partially, and may have some side effects. In other words, don't believe everything in the advertisements.

Another possible effect is that anxiety may change the response time. To say it again, anxiety affects the effectiveness of medication. Perhaps if both of you treat it as a "Well, let's see what happens" situation, anxiety will be minimized. Even if a medication is not entirely effective, if your anxiety is lessened, it may enable your natural ability to resurface, which may then be enhanced by the medication. In situations where men have erectile

Both partners must have realistic expectations if a couple agrees to use a commercial impotence therapy. The therapy may not work, may work partially, and will possibly have some side effects.

dysfunction, a percentage (generally thought to be about 10 percent) of relationships improves with any medication, primarily because performance anxiety is relieved. Often, if a couple had a satisfactory physical relationship before prostate surgery or radiation, a "starting aid" is sufficient to get over the anxiety threshold.

On the other hand, there is "anxiety override." A man concerned about whether he will have an erection and be able to perform may already know that this chronic anxiety will diminish any natural ability he has. Even when he takes a medication that could be effective, anxiety can suppress the effect of the medication.

We have provided much medical, medication and therapy, and product information, because being an informed patient/consumer is essential to good health and optimal health care. However, the information is not presented for patients to treat themselves. Patients must consult with their doctors so that informed, joint decisions can be made. Doctors have the medical background and your history to work with in order to prescribe the best approach for your health care and quality of life.

You can help your doctor and yourself in discussing treatment options by requesting product-prescribing information. This information is available in the form of package inserts. Some companies also provide a patient package insert written in "nonscientific" language.

Before we discuss medication aids for erections, we offer a word about therapies and dosages for those aids that offer a choice. Conservative treatment philosophy is:

- Begin with the least invasive therapy.

Be kind to your body—ask your doctor whether the prescribed treatment is conservative.

- In the case of drugs, start with the lowest possible dosage, see if it works, and as necessary, gradually work your way up to a higher dosage. Any medication may have side effects. A new medication may have unexpected results. This is equivalent to deciding how much whiskey to give to a person who has never had liquor before. Some people would give them half a shot, others would give them a glassful.

So try the minimum, and increase as necessary. However, this requires a supportive partner who is willing to work with you, and won't put you down if the low dosage does not work. You need to work with your doctor regarding medication dosage. Guessing at the appropriate dosage may lead to problems.

Injection medication should be "titrated" by the patient's doctor *in the office*. (Titration is the process of beginning with a certain amount of a chemical and adding known amounts until the point is reached at which the desired reaction occurs.) As an informed patient you should insist on it. If the doctor is unwilling, go elsewhere. Always try to put the least burden on your system.

Some medicines change the way other medications work. Tell your doctor about all medicines you are taking before new ones are prescribed. The prospective new medication may not be as effective or in conflict with other medications you are currently taking. The combination may worsen side effects or, in the worst case, the combination may be extremely harmful or fatal.

The following pages present currently available information on seven categories of products. We have tried to be as accurate as possible. In some cases, information was obtained from several sources. Most of the manufacturers commented on the draft material concerning their product(s). In addition, drug prices and other information were obtained from some drugstore chains and an independent pharmacy in the Baltimore/Washington area. For different reasons, some information could not be obtained, and these instances have been noted as "not available."

Unfortunately, companies with New Drug Applications pending for Food and Drug Administration (FDA) approval cannot release much information on these products. In these instances we have provided as much as we have been able to obtain. Therefore, our commentary varies from product to product. Moreover, given the rate at which new information is becoming available, you must check with your doctor to get the latest information concerning any existing or new medication or erectile dysfunction therapy.

Some of the products are in development and are noted here for information purposes only. There are probably others in the pipeline that we are not aware of.

We do not recommend or endorse any product. Also because of possible contraindications (adverse reactions) and new information becoming available continually, any piece of information could become quickly outdated. Additionally, an individual's response to a medication is a function of many factors, including body weight, genetics, and physiology. Therefore, you should not use the following information as a basis for any medical decision.

The prices noted are only provided as a reference point. Prices will differ depending on area of the country, the pharmacy, and other conditions. Before you buy, it is okay to ask your pharmacy about price and what proportion is covered by insurance.

Oral Medications/Treatments

In mid-1998, many men found a new deity, the goddess Viagra. The impact of this pill was rather well expressed in a urologist's Christmas letter we received "John's year has been dominated by that little blue pill, Viagra."

Viagra (said to be named after Robert Virag, who reported on means for producing erections in 1982), approved in mid-1998, was the first pill for erectile dysfunction to reach the market. Several other pills are being developed and will be introduced after expected approval in the last half of 1999 and early 2000. In contrast to Viagra, which works on the penis, a product being developed by TAP Pharmaceuticals works on chemicals in the brain that initiate erections.

A key point for many medications is the comment that Pfizer issues for Viagra: "These drugs do not increase desire. All they do is help a man who already has the desire for sex to achieve an erection." This statement applies to all known oral medications. So if you become "turned off," you will lose the erection.

No oral erection medication is intended to be administered or taken several times a day. Also they should not be used every day.

No pill will enable a man to have an orgasm. Also, none of these drugs facilitate repeated orgasms. As we get older, the period between orgasms increases, and the ability to have orgasms decreases. However, Viagra is reported to make it easier to have an orgasm.

The primary erectile oral product available today is Pfizer's prescription drug, Viagra, whose effectiveness is well documented. The other prescription oral product is yohimbine, which has debatable capability. We are aware of three other oral medications that are in development and/or clinical trials.

The following pages present currently available information on these products. The products are presented in alphabetical order by manufacturer in two parts. First are the currently available products, followed by those under development. Yohimbine is listed under its generic name (following Viagra) because there are many manufacturers.

Manufacturer: Pfizer
Brand Name: Viagra
Active Chemical: Sildenafil citrate in tablet form.
Dosage: Dosage: 25 mg, 50 mg, 100 mg
Administration: The maximum dose that can be taken in one day is 100 mg. The pill must be taken on an empty stomach (at least two hours after a meal), and after taking the pill you should wait about 1 hour before lovemaking. A low-fat meal is best. Food and fat delay and reduce intestinal absorption, thereby reducing the drug's effectiveness. The man should not use alcohol when taking Viagra. The drug will take effect within 30-60 minutes in most patients. The erectile effects of the drug may last up to four hours.
Status: Available since April 1998
Price: $8–$9 per pill regardless of dosage
Side Effects: Major caution is that Viagra must not be taken if you are taking nitrate medication, or have unstable cardiac disease. This information has been extensively publicized. Most of the 138 fatalities associated with taking the drug in 1998 were in patients taking Viagra who disregarded the warnings about the drug's conflict with nitrate medication. Therefore, if you take any nitrate medication, even if prescribed only on an "as needed" basis, you should not be using Viagra.

An additional safety concern that is sometimes overlooked by this patient population is their ability to safely engage in sexual activity with or without Viagra therapy. Many men in our generation, especially those with multiple underlying disease problems, may not have been engaging in any regular physical activity (and probably not in sex). Now, with the potential for them to again engage in sexual relations because of Viagra therapy, they should be evaluated by their doctor to determine their ability to tolerate the physical exertion that is part of any sexual activity. As the Pfizer patient summary puts it, "ask your doctor if your heart is healthy enough to handle the extra strain of having sex. If you have chest pains, dizziness, or nausea during sex, stop having sex and immediately call your doctor. . . ."

The most publicized side effect is a blue-green haze and increased perception of bright light several hours after taking Viagra that affected 3 percent of patients in the clinical trials. This effect was reported more frequently at the higher dose of 100 mg.

Other side effects include headache (16 percent) (similar to coital headaches), stomach upset or nausea (11 percent), facial flushing (7 percent), abdominal pains, and some sinus difficulty including nasal congestion.

Comments: Men should begin with a low dosage, and try it three times (not in one day nor on three consecutive days) before discussing increasing the dosage with their doctor. Viagra improves erections and is reported to enhance orgasm.

Study results have shown that it was effective in 43 percent of radical prostatectomy patients. Effectiveness is supposedly better for radiation patients. Patients taking Lupron can have erections with Viagra and so can orchiectomy patients.

Viagra is also prescribed in combination with the vacuum pump and/or constriction rings such as Actis.

As previously mentioned, no erection will occur unless you are aroused. Taking the pill and reading the newspaper until there is an erection means that you are in for a long reading session. It will not happen. Similarly, if you are aroused and have an erection, but are suddenly distracted or think about how your stocks went down that day, so will the erection. However, since the effects of the drug may last for up to four hours-that is, a man has the capability for an erection for that time-if there is a low moment, the couple can try later on. There is no guidance on how many times in one week Viagra may be used. Moderation as always is the key, and following the guidance of the manufacturers who make injection medication, a maximum of three times seems like a good guideline.

For more information: Pfizer Corporation
Tel: 888-4VIAGRA.
Website: www.viagra.com

Reader's Notes:

Manufacturer: ICOS Corporation
Brand Name: Not available
Active Chemical: Photodiesterase type 5 inhibitors (PDE-5)
Dosage: Information not available
Administration: Orally
Status: In development
Price: Not available
Side Effects: Information not available
Comments: In October 1998, Eli Lilly and ICOS Corporation announced that they decided to form a 50/50 joint venture to develop and globally commercialize this oral therapeutic agent for treatment of male and female sexual dysfunction. The product is in the early stage of development.
For more information:
Tel: 206-485-1900.
Website: www.icos.com

Reader's Notes:

Manufacturer: TAP Pharmaceuticals
Brand Name: Uprima
Active Chemical: Apomorphine
Dosage: Not available
Administration: The pill is to be taken sublingually (dissolved under the tongue).
Status: Applied for FDA approval
Price: Not available
Side Effects: The major side effect is likely to be some yawning and possibly some nausea because apomorphine is an emetic (causes vomiting).
Comments: Uprima, a dopamine agonist, is designed to work in the central nervous system, using the body's natural pathways to produce an erection. It stimulates the brain center for sexual response, which then transmits the message down the spinal cord to produce an erection. The drug is designed to work on men with mild to moderate erectile dysfunction.

Data from three Phase III clinical trials reported at the 1999 American Urological Association (AUA) meeting showed that Uprima "can increase the number of successful intercourse attempts." The studies used four dosage levels. The level of successful intercourse increased from 44 percent of the men at the lowest dosage, 2 mg., to 61 percent at 4 mg. The company also reported that the most common side effect was mild to moderate nausea.

Additional trials have been initiated or will soon be conducted in about 150 centers in the United States and Canada. TAP is focusing its clinical trials on studying the drug's safety and efficacy in helping men with diabetes and prostate surgery cope with erectile dysfunction. Information provided at the AUA conference in 1998 indicated that patients must have an intact vascular system.

One formulation of Uprima has been shown to cause erections without visual or manual stimulation. However, it is not known if this is the formulation the company is developing for commercial use.

In July 1999, TAP Pharmaceuticals (a joint venture between Abbott Laboratories and Takeda) announced it had filed a New Drug Application with the FDA. On this basis, drug approval was expected in late 1999, or early 2000.

For more information:
Tel: 800-348-2779.
Website: www.tapurology.com

Reader's Notes:

Manufacturer: Zonagen
Brand Name: Vasomax
Active Chemical: Phentolamine—an alpha blocker, opens the blood vessels in the vascular smooth muscles of the penis to help restore normal function in approximately 15 minutes with normal sexual stimulation.
Dosage: Information not available
Administration: Information not available
Status: Applied for FDA approval
Price: Not available
Side Effects: Not available
Comments: The company has filed a new drug application for FDA approval and is therefore precluded from providing any current information. Previously available information showed that in a 148-patient Phase II clinical trial in Mexico, the drug worked on 42 percent of the men in every attempt. Two U.S. Phase III trials showed improvement in 34 percent and 40 percent of the men. There were some circulatory side effects. Zonagen is currently conducting additional, large open-label studies with Vasomax.

Phentolamine has been around for a long time, and its effectiveness has been disputed. Its effectiveness is apparently due to its being a combined alpha-1 and alpha-2 blocker. Its current formulation permits the body to absorb it, whereas the body did not retain other formulations.

Zonagen licensed worldwide marketing rights to the product to Schering Plough in October 1998.

In August 1999, the Food and Drug Administration (FDA) placed further clinical trials of Zonagen's phentolamine-based drugs (including Vasomax) on hold until "issues surrounding the Company's two-year rat study are satisfactorily resolved. FDA is allowing Schering-Plough [Vasomax licensee] to complete the . . . ongoing 12-week study in humans of Vasomax for erectile dysfunction."

For more information: Company does not wish to be contacted while drug is under FDA review. Website: www.zonagen.com

Reader's Notes:

Active Chemical: Yohimbine
Manufacturer: Many, e.g., Duramed, Palisades Pharmaceutical and others
Brand Name: Actibine, Aphrodyne, Baron-X, Dayto Himbin, PMS-Yohimbine, Prohim, Thybine, Yocon, Yohlmar, Yohimex, Yoman, Yovital
Dosage: Each tablet contains 5.4 mg. yohimbine.
Administration: 1 tablet 2–4 times daily
Status: Available with prescription only. (Yohimbine is a controlled substance.)
Price: Varies
Side Effects: Anxiety, increase in blood pressure, nervousness
Comments: Yohimbine has been rumored to be an aphrodisiac for many years. While it has been shown to be "highly effective in castrated rats, several clinical studies have shown only moderate success in men. . . ." The chemical seems more effective in patients with psychologically based impotence than in those with an organic basis. "Despite these relatively poor results, yohimbine is often prescribed . . . because of its relatively mild side effects. . . ."

Results of studies conflict. One study concluded that the benefits of using yohimbine outweigh the risks and suggested that it "remain a viable option for men with erectile dysfunction." (*Journal of Urology*, July 1998.) A paper presented at the 1998 American Urological Association (AUA) meeting quotes "the recent AUA guidelines for erectile dysfunction suggest that this drug is little better than a placebo."

Although yohimbine sales are high, that does not mean it works. Ineffective substances often have the greatest sales when there is a perception that they have minimal side effects.

For more information: Search for Yohimbine on the Internet

Reader's Notes:

Topical Medications: Penile Creams and Gels

Topical medications include gels and creams that are applied directly to the head or the glans of the penis. We are aware that three gels-that is, Vaseline-type or creamlike products-are in development. The competitive advantage offered by topical medications is that they "could offer doctors a safer alternative to oral pills," which have a whole-body (systemic) effect. Because they are easy to use, this class of products may be a more acceptable alternative to injections and Muse. In the course of developing these products, due diligence demands that companies also investigate possible effects on partners. None of the products are currently available.

The following products are presented in alphabetical order by manufacturer.

Manufacturer: Harvard Scientific Corporation
Brand Name: Not available
Active Chemical: Prostaglandin E-1
Dosage: Information not available
Administration: Topically applied gel, topically applied liquid spray, or an aqueous (liquid) solution administered into the urethra via a small applicator tip.
Status: In development and clinical trials
Price: Not available
Side Effects: Information not available
Comments: The company's core technology is covered by U.S. patent no. 5,718,917 for "PGE1 containing lyophilized liposomes for use in the treatment of erectile dysfunction." Prostaglandin E-1 is the same chemical used in Caverject and Muse.
For more information:
Tel: 775-323-6751.
Website: www.harvardscientific.com

Reader's Notes:

Manufacturer: MacroChem
Brand Name: Topiglan
Active Chemical: Alprostadil
Dosage: Not available
Administration: This is a topical gel formulation of alprostadil that is applied directly on the end surface of the penis to induce an erection and "is user-friendly." The gel is absorbed by the penis through the skin by SEPA, a patented absorption enhancer. The company's SEPA technology modifies layers in the skin, allowing the compounds to be absorbed. Stimulation increases the effectiveness of the medication.
Status: In development and clinical trials
Price: Not available
Side Effects: Information not available
Comments: Gel applied directly to the penis is considered local therapy in contrast to the whole-body systemic therapy provided by oral medications such as Viagra. Based on positive Phase I and II clinical trials, the company has accelerated its development program. The product is noninvasive (no injection required) and is a non-systemic approach (no pill). About 67–75 percent of patients responded to the topical therapy. This gel does not contain testosterone. Testosterone is a concern for prostate cancer patients and is a component of MacroChem's other topical product. In June 1998, Dr. Irwin Goldstein said that the AUA recommended the company begin a multicenter, double-blind Phase III study.

In February 1999, the U.S. Patent and Trademark Office issued a "Notice of Allowance" (approving the company's product claims) of all claims covering the company's Topiglan topical formulation for the treatment of male erectile dysfunction.
For more information:
Tel: 781-862-4003
Website: www. mchm.com or www.macrochem.com

Reader' Notes:

Manufacturer: NexMed Inc.
Brand Name: Alprox-TD
Active Chemical: Alprostadil (prostaglandin E-1)
Dosage: Information not available
Administration: Topical cream is applied directly onto the tip of the penis at least 15 minutes before intercourse from a novel, easy-to-use single-dose applicator. Rapid absorption is obtained using the patented NexACT skin penetration enhancement technology
Status: In clinical trials. Approval is expected in two foreign countries in 1999.
Price: Not available
Side Effects: Information not available
Comments: The product is in various stages of clinical testing throughout the world. In double-blind, placebo controlled Phase III, multicenter, clinical studies conducted in China, the product had an overall efficacy rate of 75 percent with minimal side effects.

Clinical studies have shown that the product works within 15-20 minutes after application, but it could be applied up to one hour before intercourse, making it a versatile product. No spousal side effects have been reported with Alprox-TD.

NexMed is also developing a female version of the drug, Femprox. Phase I trials have been satisfactorily completed. Phase II trials will be initiated shortly.

For more information:
Tel: 609-208-9688.
Website: www.nexmedinc.com

Reader's Notes:

Devices

Vacuum pumps and penile splints are generally considered noninvasive, although some doctors consider pumps as minimally invasive.

Penile Splints and Supports

A prosthesis is basically a penile splint that supports the penis in penetration. These splints have been available in adult stores for a long time.

In 1996, American MedTech introduced its first product, a penile support sleeve called "Rejoyn." This is a variant of the old penile splint. The company's material states: "Rejoyn is designed to enable a man with a flaccid penis to engage in intercourse."

Rejoyn is a "patented penile support sleeve . . . made of high grade, natural feeling Santoprene (neoprene) rubber" that fits around the penis. The support sleeve is held in place by a condomlike sheath. The front part of the sheath is cut off to permit penile sensation.

The stiffness of the neoprene provides the support. We've been told that the woman needs to control movement; otherwise, the penile support could hurt her.

For further information, call the American MedTech Corporation at 1-800-578-7358, or visit their website at www.rejoyn.com.

Vacuum Pumps

Vacuum devices, also known as pumps, have been around for about 25 years and currently are estimated to have over 500,000 users. Doctors frequently prescribe them because they are relatively safe, provide immediate results, and are noninvasive. This type of device creates a vacuum using some type of actuating mechanism.

Vacuum devices consist of a cylinder, vacuum pump (manual or battery-operated), constriction rings, and water-based lubricant. The steps for using a vacuum pump consist of:

1. Connecting the vacuum pump to the cylinder.

2. Lubricating the penis and placing it inside the cylinder.

3. Positioning the cylinder firmly against the body to form an airtight seal.

4. Activating the vacuum pump to remove air from the cylinder. This creates negative pressure and causes blood to be drawn into the penis to create an erection.

5. A constriction ring is then placed at the base of the penis to maintain the erection. If a constriction ring is not used, the blood will flow back into the body and the erection will be lost.

There are some differences between a natural erection and one created by a vacuum device:

- The penis may become "cool" after a short period because the constriction ring decreases blood flow to the penis.

- The penis may be bigger around and longer than with a natural erection because all the tissues of the penis beyond the constriction ring are filled with blood. The penis may appear darker, and the veins will stand out.

- There is little vertical control of the penis. The penis may pivot at the base because it is rigid only beyond the constriction point. In a natural erection, hardness extends back into the body. However, after penetration has been accomplished, the "pivot effect" or the "hinge effect," as it is sometimes called, does not interfere with intercourse.

Several sexual dysfunction specialists noted that erectile success with a pump is about 98 percent even though a common complaint is that pumps are a lot of fuss. Despite the foregoing effects, and possibly some loss of sensitivity, long-term satisfaction is about 70–75%. One specialist noted that about half the dropouts go on to implants.

To our knowledge, six companies manufacture vacuum devices. The inventor of the modern-day vacuum treatment for impotence, Geddings Osbon, founded the first company to make pumps, Osbon Medical Systems.

Osbon was acquired in 1998 by Timm Medical Technologies. The company has three ErecAid products that sell at prices of $395, $425, and $475, respectively. They can be obtained with a doctor's prescription or through designated retail outlets. There is also an over-the-counter ErecAid classic device that is available without a prescription. For further information, call Timm Medical Systems at 1-800-438-8592.

Other vacuum pump companies are American Medtech, Encore, Mission Pharmacal, Pos-T-Vac, and Vetco. American MedTech is also the manufacturer of the Rejoyn penile splint. The company's Rejoyn vacuum therapy device is sold in drug stores such as CVS. In early 1999, the price in the Washington, DC area was about $150.

Caution: One vacuum device is not the same as another. Since use of such devices creates physical and to some extent physiological changes in the penis, you should use a device only with care. Your particular situation may make it advisable to consult a urologist or sexual dysfunction specialist. Your partner should be included in the discussions because you must work together in using this aid.

Recently, the FDA approved some vacuum devices for sale without prescription. Nevertheless, Medicare and many private insurance plans continue to reimburse patients for prescribed vacuum devices. If you intend to use a vacuum device, a doctor's prescription should be obtained even if you plan to purchase an over-the-counter model because you may be eligible for reimbursement.

A cautionary note: On September 10, 1997, the FDA issued an Interim Regulatory Policy guideline for external rigidity devices. The guideline specified a maximum safe vacuum limit of 17 inches of mercury (440 millimeters of mercury). Make sure that any vacuum device you purchase meets this safety requirement.

Manufacturers of Erectile Dysfunction Devices

American MedTech
Rejoyn penile splints
Rejoyn vacuum pumps
  2124 University Avenue
  St. Paul, MN 55114
  Tel: 888-209-8609
      651-659-2406
  Web: www.rejoyn.com

Encore Medical Products Inc.
Encore vacuum pumps
  1002 North Central Expressway
  Suite 341
  Richardson, TX 75080
  Tel: 800-221-6603
  email: encoreved@aol.com

Mentor
Sold its vacuum pump line to Vetco
  Tel: 800-328-3863

Mission Pharmacal
VED vacuum pumps
  10999 IH-10 West Suite 1000
  San Antonio, TX 78230-1355
      or
  PO Box 786099
  San Antonio, TX 78278-6099
  Tel: 800-292-7364
  Web: www.missionpharmacal.com

Pos-T-Vac
IVP vacuum pumps
  1701 North 14th Avenue
  P.O. Box 1436
  Dodge City, KS 67801
  Tel: 800-279-7434
  Web: www.postvac.com

Timm Medical
Osbon vacuum pumps
  6585 City West Parkway
  Eden Prairie, MN 55344
  Tel: 800-438-8592
  Web: www.erectionsolutions.com

Vetco Inc.
Vetco and Mentor vacuum pumps
  3700th Avenue S
  Birmingham, AL 35222
  Tel: 800-827-8382
  Web: www.vetcoinc.com

Intraurethral Medication

Intraurethral medication consists of drugs that are inserted directly into the urethra, the opening in the penis. One intraurethral medication, Muse is currently available. Muse is a suppository medication, in the form of a cylinder, that is inserted into the penis with a penile syringe. This tubelike device enables the user to place the suppository far enough into the penis for it to take effect. Erections occur in about 15 minutes.

Manufacturer: VIVUS, Inc.
Brand Name: Muse
Active Chemical: Alprostadil
Dosage: Four dosage levels: 125, 250, 500, and 1000 micrograms
Administration: The first treatment should be under medical supervision. The medication in the form of a pellet is delivered to the urethral membrane by an applicator, which is inserted into the opening of the penis. The man should urinate immediately prior to insertion. The few drops of urine remaining in the urethra lubricate the urinary tract in the penis and make it easier to insert the stem of the Muse applicator. Do not use Vaseline or any type of oil or grease as a lubricant because it may interfere with the absorption of the pellet.

To eliminate or at least minimize pain, the penis should be pulled out and upward in order to straighten the urethra prior to inserting the stem of the applicator. The applicator should be inserted slowly and carefully, and withdrawn if resistance is felt. The man should try to insert the applicator again after further straightening the penis. The man is cautioned to insert the applicator slowly.
Status: Available
Price: $100 per box of six doses, about 80-85 percent covered by insurance
Side Effects: Intraurethral administration may be psychologically easier than injection. The most common side effect is penile pain which is due to the effects of alprostadil being inserted. About one-third of the men in the clinical trial experienced penile pain. Discomfort gradually decreased after multiple administrations.
Comments: A man who fails to respond to injectable medication, may still find Muse effective. One study reported that 58 percent of the patients who did not respond to injections "achieved an erection satisfactory for intercourse after Muse in the clinic, and 50 percent of these responsive patients continued to use Muse successfully for intercourse at home" (*International Journal of Impotence Research* 8(3):146,1996).

One physician said that he routinely begins his patients at 500 mcg at home, increasing to 1,000 mcg if the erection response is insufficient. Men considering using Muse should not become dejected if it does not work. As noted previously, no medication will work on everyone.

VIVUS is reported to be researching the effectiveness of intraurethral alprostadil in combination with other vasoactive agents.

Although Muse may get blood into the penis to cause an erection, it can only be maintained if the blood remains in the penis. Many patients with erectile dysfunction also have an associated disorder of the veno-occlusive mechanism called venous leak syndrome.

This condition results in the failure to retain blood within the penis. Venous leakage prevents the storage of blood and therefore an erection cannot be maintained. In July 1997, VIVUS introduced a venous flow controller, Actis, which is the only approved adjustable band for use with Muse. It is placed at the base of the penis for treatment of venous leak syndrome. The product works to diminish systemic absorption and enhance the erectile effect of Muse by retaining more alprostadil in the penis and preventing blood from flowing out of the penis. The use of Muse plus Actis is currently under clinical investigation in the U.S. In August 1998, Vivus presented research data on the efficacy of Muse (alprostadil) when used together with Actis, showing that, during home treatment, 75 percent of administrations of the combination resulted in sexual intercourse. Erections lasted approximately 25 minutes. The average study patient had moderate to complete erectile dysfunction.

For more information:
Tel: 888-367-6873
Website: www.vivus.com

Reader's Notes:

Penile Injection

Most of the work that led to injections began about 15 years ago with Robert Virag's studies on the effect of papaverine. The results were such that by the end of 1998 there were at least six injection products and compounds available. This array enabled physicians to address the needs of patients as they concerned effectiveness, penile pain, and other side effects.

A key precondition for using any injectable medication is that the man must be willing to insert a needle into his penis. Most men find that the biggest problem with the needle is the apprehension leading up to its use. Many men feel queasy. However, when the needle is inserted correctly, quickly, and from the side of the penis (at the 2 or 10 o'clock position), a man should feel no more than a nanosecond pinprick in the skin of the penis, much like pinching his earlobe or the skin on his elbow. Some men have found it acceptable for their partner to administer the injection.

Although injection works without stimulation, the penis will be more rigid with stimulation.

The key benefits of injection are:

- The erection occurs within 5–15 minutes.

- The man will have increased stamina/sustainability.

- It is highly effective-injection produces an erection in most cases.

The primary disadvantage is penile pain from the injection and from the medication, experienced by about 37 percent of the men in one clinical trial. In addition, in less than 10 percent of men, injection medication can lead to fibrosis that creates scars that impair the delivery of blood to the penis, which worsens erectile dysfunction.

Injection therapy demands close doctor-patient cooperation. The doctor must:

1. determine the dosage by beginning with an initiation dose and observing the effect. This is done in the physician's office.

2. ensure that you are properly trained in administering the injection.

3. observe that there are no severe complications and address any complications that occur.

The doctor's objective is to make sure that you are able to do penile injections at home safely and with the desired effect.

An injection can have serious and even fatal side effects if the erection lasts too long (priapism). If the injection is done properly, a priapism should be a rare event. Caverject labeling approved by the FDA specifies that erections lasting four hours or longer should be treated. The man should seek immediate treatment if an erection lasts four hours. The medication required to end the erection is similar to that used for asthma or high blood pressure. As a precautionary measure, men using injections are advised to have a medication at hand such as phenylephrine, ephedrine, norepinephrine, or epinephrine. We understand that an over-the counter nasal decongestant such as Breathin will work as well. Before taking any over-the-counter products, as well as any other medications, patients should consult their physician.

Now we will describe three penile injection products and three blends that doctors may prepare for particular erectile dysfunction cases.

Any of the medications discussed in this section may be administered with less discomfort by using the Osbon InjectAid System. In this system, the design of the injection tip helps reduce sensitivity at the point of injection. The delivery system has an automatic release for a quick, yet smooth injection. Injection discomfort is minimized and simplified because it uses Becton Dickinson 1-cc insulin syringes with smaller-gauge needles than may be used for penile injections. Kits may be ordered from Osbon ($48.75 per kit for up to three kits.) Each kit includes 10 syringes and needles.

Men who experience pain with injected medication should be aware that the pain is due primarily to the prostaglandin E-1 (alprostadil). The pain results from the way the prostaglandin is absorbed through the membrane. About 50 percent of the users experience some pain; only 10–20 percent have severe pain. We know of a doctor who prescribes lidocaine with the injection medication to lessen and, in some cases, eliminate the pain.

For some patients, combinations of active ingredients have been responsible for better erectile responses than any ingredient alone. These combinations are shown at the end of this section. A *World of Urology* 1997 article noted response rates in studies that exceeded 90 percent. One study using a four-drug combination in 94 patients resulted in a response rate of 96 percent. Any man considering taking any injection medication should explore with his doctor the prospective downsides. Some discomfort accompanies all injections.

Manufacturer: Pharmacia/Upjohn
Brand Name: Caverject
Active Chemical: Alprostadil
Dosage: Three alternative formulations:
Sterile powder vials: 5, 10, 20, and 40 mcg
Sterile powder kits: 5, 10, and 20 mcg
Aqueous solution: 10, 20, and 40 mcg
Administration: Note: The medication should not be used more than three times a week. Men must allow at least twenty-four hours to elapse between successive injections.

The user first mixes the liquid and powder. Then the volume of medication is extracted from the vial for injection into the penis. The product and technique for administration is safe with proper training. First-time users must be taught how to administer injections by a doctor or qualified health professional. As noted previously, the patient and doctor must work together to determine the appropriate dosage.
Status: Available.
Price: A Washington-area pharmacy charges $140.99, $176.99, and $185.99 for six-packs of the three dosages. This works out to $23.50, $29.50, and $31.00 per shot for the three dosages, respectively. Generally, the price for the 10-mcg aqueous solution is $164-180 for a six-pack ; for the 20-mcg aqueous solution, $185–190.
Side Effects: The major complaint is penile pain, which is the direct effect of the medication, not the injection. Discomfort is a function of the dosage, and ranges from a dull ache to burning pain. During the clinical trials, the company reports about 37 percent of the patients had penile pain. Severe pain is experienced by 10-20 percent of men. Fibrosis (forming of little nodules in the penis) is a concern.
Comments: According to Upjohn, this medication is indicated when the cause for erectile dysfunction is due to neurological, vascular, or psychological problems, as well as mixed causes. This includes the typical prostate cancer-related causes. It should not

be used when the man has conditions that could lead to prolonged erections (priapism). According to one erectile dysfunction specialist, there is less risk of priapism with Caverject than with other injectables.

The company recently introduced the new aqueous (water-based) formulation to supplement the existing products. This product is available in pre-mixed, single-use, plastic ampoules, and is therefore ready for injection preparation. Key benefits are that it is easier to use, and sterility, quality, and consistency are assured. Since it is reconstituted, the product must be stored in the freezer and has a limited shelf life of three months. Users should read the special handling instructions.

The company also now offers a thinner 30-gauge needle in addition to the standard 27-gauge needle. Previously, injection patients resorted to the often recommended Osbon diabetic syringe with its smaller needle diameter because it minimizes injection discomfort.

For more information:
Tel: 800-253-8600.
Website: www.impotent.com

Reader's Notes:

Manufacturer: Schwarz Pharma
Trade Name: Edex
Active Chemical: Alprostadil
Dosage: Edex cartridges are supplied in strengths of 10, 20, and 40 mcg. The product should not be used more than 3 times per week and there should be at least 24 hours between each dose.
Administration: EDEX is available in two forms: (1) as a powder that must be mixed with the saline solution provided in a kit, and (2) as a cartridge where the solution and powder are in one container. In both instances, the cartridge is placed in the reusable EDEX injection device that is used to reconstitute the sterile powder. EDEX is given as an intracavernous injection over a 5- to 10- second interval. As with all injections, drops or solutions should not be added to the product provided by the manufacturer.
Status: Available. Prescription only. Introduced June 1997
Price: $120-135 for 4 shots of the 20 mcg and $169-185 for 4 shots of the 40mcg dosage.
Side Effects: About 41 percent of patients had penile pain which decreased over time. Some patients experienced prolonged erections. Fibrosis is also a concern.
Comments: EDEX is indicated for the treatment of erectile dysfunction due to neurological, vascular, psychological, or mixed causes.

EDEX should not be used in patients who are sensitive to the active chemical alprostadil or any other prostaglandins, or in patients who have conditions that might increase the possibility of priapism (prolonged erection), such as sickle-cell anemia, multiple myeloma, or anatomical deformations of the penis. Patients with penile implants should not be treated with EDEX.

Schwarz provides 29-gauge needles for injection as standard. The company also provides an optional, thinner 30-gauge needle with kits to minimize injection discomfort.

A comparison of EDEX versus MUSE was presented at the 8th World Meeting on Impotence Research in August 1998. The results, based on in-office data, showed that Schwarz's intracavernous alprostadil-alfadex (EDEX/VIRIDAL) combination had a statistically significant higher efficacy and safety than did MUSE plus the use of the ACTIS device, both produced by VIVUS.

For more information:
Tel: 414-354-4300.
Website: www.edex.com

Reader's Notes:

Manufacturer: Senetek
Trade Name: Invicorp
Active Chemical: Vasoactive intestinal polypeptide in combination with the adrenergic drug phentolamine mesylate (PMS)
Dosage: Information not available
Administration: Proprietary state-of-the-art autoinjector
Status: Not available in the US. Available in Denmark and possibly in the United Kingdom (See Comments).
Price: Not available
Side Effects: Penile pain from the injection and from the medication was experienced by about 37 percent of the men in one clinical trial. In addition, the medication can lead to fibrosis, which impairs the delivery of blood to the penis.
Comments: In March 1999, the United Kingdom's Committee on Safety of Medicines of the Medicines Control Agency decided to advise the Licensing Authority to authorize the marketing of Senetek's Invicorp new drug therapy for treating moderate to severe, organic-based erectile dysfunction. The company expects full marketing authorization. In 1998, the Danish Medicine Agency approved Invicorp for the treatment of moderate to severe erectile dysfunction.

In clinical studies published in the March 1999 issue of the *British Journal of Urology*, Invicorp proved effective in 82 percent of patients. In another study, the company noted that 59 percent of the patients treated successfully with Invicorp "had previously been treated with alternative pharmacotherapies, including prostaglandin, papaverine and yohimbine but had withdrawn from treatment either due to lack of effectiveness or side effects."
For more information:
Tel: 800-758-5804.
Website: www.senetekpic.com

Reader's Notes:

Manufacturer: Individual doctors prescribing their own mixes

Brand Name: No brand name because doctors prepare their own compounds; hence the label "blends."

Active Chemical: Injectable medications come in basic combinations, as well as in what is known as bi-mix, tri-mix, and even quad-mix. Specifically, these combinations are:

1. **bi-mix**: papaverine-phentolamine (better than papaverine alone)

2. **tri-mix**: papaverine-phentolamine-prostaglandin E-1

3. **quad-mix**: forskolin-papaverine-phentolamine-prostaglandin E-1

Dosage: Varies by patient

Administration: Penile injection

Status: Prepared by local doctor

Price: Pharmacy price is approximately $150-$250 for 20 shots, depending on dosage.

Side Effects: Penile pain, fibrosis

Comments:

   Tri-mix: In one study, the tri-mix worked in 62 percent of the patients who had failed to respond to other injections. Some men had penile pain.

   Quad-mix: This product was developed for men on whom tri-mix did not work. In one study comparing tri-mix and quad-mix, the inclusion of forskolin in quad-mix "resulted in substantial improvements in rigidity and duration, 47 percent vs. 80 percent rigidity and 20 mins. vs. 67 mins." (*Journal of Urology* 155(5)A743, 996).

For more information: Contact your own physician or pharmacy.

Reader's Notes:

Penile Implants

A penile implant is a mechanical device that enables an erection. It is surgically implanted to handle the problem of erectile dysfunction. Implants were more widely recommended as the solution of choice for erectile dysfunction prior to the introduction of injections and other recent medications. Many men elect to have this procedure when available medication is not effective.

Implants can last eight to 20 years. Some implant procedures are performed as minor outpatient surgery. However, one survivor reported that surgery for a semirigid required a two-day hospital stay. He noted it was "*tough* surgery. Recovery was longer than for my radical prostatectomy."

There are three forms of implants:

Semirigid-Malleable: Hard silicon with a rod in the center. Implant is "worn" bent down and is straightened for intercourse.

- Advantage: This implant is a simple device and not likely to fail for mechanical reasons.

- Disadvantages: The implant is rigid all the time and is not cosmetically natural.

Semirigid-Positionable

- Advantage: More positionable/controllable due to hinge mechanism.

- Implant is more concealable and is more rigid.

Inflatable: There are three types:

2-component with reservoir in scrotum

3-component with reservoir in the abdomen

3-component with pump in the scrotum

- Advantages: Cosmetically, the product looks natural. The implant is concealed nicely in swim trunks and gym clothes.

- Disadvantage: The key problems that may lead to device replacement are device malfunction, infection, and pain. Replacements must be done surgically.

Penile Vascular Surgery

Vascular surgery in the penis consists of two procedures. One is called *penile revascularization*, which consists of inserting blood vessels to carry blood into the penis because the existing ones can no longer perform the function. "The overall goal of penile vascularization surgery is to bypass an obstructive arterial lesion" in the main penile arteries. The circulation of the penis is complex, so the primary candidates are young men who have had an injury.

The surgery takes about six hours. Complications may include uncontrolled bleeding in the penis during the first few weeks after surgery, pain in the penis, and diminished sensation. Also, the surgery may cause a shortening of the penis.

The other procedure is venous ligation which cuts off some of the veins that carry blood out of the penis, and thereby puts the vascular system in balance. However, survivors indicate that this does not work very well or for very long. These procedures only work when erectile dysfunction results from simple vascular injury. It is usually not an option for prostate cancer patients who have had surgery or radiation.

Commercial Therapies and Medications

Key Points

When using any of these commercial therapies, remember:

- There are many different types of aids for erectile dysfunction.
- The physician must be involved to determine dosage, train and observe you using the technique, and address possible complications.
- Each aid has its own advantages and drawbacks and problems, and may not work for you. Don't get frustrated if something does not work; try something else. It's also very important that the partner have realistic expectations in case a medication does not work.
- If possible, start with a low dosage and work your way up as necessary. This puts less burden on your system.

Chapter 6
Putting it all
Together

A ll beginnings are hard. If you have trouble figuring out how to get started, maybe the examples of the following couples will give you some ideas. As always, you have to adjust the strategy to the participants, so it depends on what kind of a relationship you and your partner have, and what your personalities are.

We'll introduce you to two couples. The first couple had been married for 26 years and had always been very romantic. Loving was very important to both partners. We'll call them Romeo and Juliet, although they are a bit older than Shakespeare's lovers.

Before Romeo had surgery, he and Juliet talked about the fact that no matter what his level of potency was, they would find a way to make love afterward. So they both knew the other was interested. After surgery, Romeo lost most of his erectile capability.

They decided to use this as an opportunity to rediscover each other. They agreed that they both would learn together and try new things, knowing that some things would work and some wouldn't. They started over, as if they were new lovers, getting to know each other's bodies all over again. They consciously slowed down the pace of their lovemaking and found that it became a completely different experience-one they liked very much! They began to read passages from books to each other, which at least one of them found erotic. They got some good laughs when they discovered that they didn't always agree on what was erotic-but most of the time they did. They also tried shots and Viagra and continue to use them, but only on "special occasions." They're using more variety in their sex life: where they make love, oral sex, manual stimulation, and lots of sensual touching.

The results? Juliet says, "I used to get frustrated sometimes because Romeo was so goal-oriented. I always wanted much more touching and sensuality. Most people would shake their heads in disbelief if I told them that now I've got everything I wanted-but it's true! I enjoy lovemaking much more now and really feel that Romeo has become an even better lover than before. We've always had a good and healthy relationship, but now I feel that our relationship is even deeper. And lovemaking is even more important to us now than it had been in the last few years."

Romeo echoes her feelings: "I was not happy when I realized that this capability that I used to think of as an essential part of me was drastically reduced. Not making love was never an option for us-whatever it took, we would do it together. But I thought that she would get most of the pleasure, and it would be mostly frustration and disappointment for me. It really hasn't happened that way. We make better love today than we ever have. I've learned things about my body and hers that I wish I'd known thirty years ago. We've found some pretty nifty places and ways to touch each other that send us both into orbit. Don't get me wrong: there are times when we both really miss the old no-fuss erections. So sometimes we use Caverject or Viagra, but that's like a special treat. And most of the time we're very happy with our unaided lovemaking. With the aids, you just tend to do the same two or three things. Without them, you let your imagination take you wherever it will. It's amazing how many different things you'll come up with."

Our second couple had a very traditional relationship and rather conservative sexual habits. Since he's a military man, we'll call them Napoleon and Josephine. Napoleon was devastated when he realized his potency was affected. He withdrew and didn't even mention sex for eight months. Josephine went on a slow but steady campaign to show her love and support and rebuild his confidence, but it took quite a while.

While giving Napoleon a massage because he seemed "so tense," Josephine found that he was okay with (nonsexual) touching. She finally figured out how to talk to him about this topic: she'd play on his military background.

She presented the enemy: absence of lovemaking due to impotence. His key ally: Josephine. His strengths: coming up with a strategy and a battle plan, and executing it with persistence.

Their challenge: Napoleon's treatment had been like an earthquake to his body. It had changed the terrain. The first step was to explore the terrain. Josephine is a very creative and convincing lady, and Napoleon bought into the idea of the plan. It included, of course, a communication plan (you must always talk to each other) and a contract: absolutely no putting down of the partner if something they tried did not work. There would be heavy penalties if the contract was broken: If she broke it, she'd have to attend a hockey game with him, and if he broke it, he'd have to accompany her to the mall while she shopped for clothes.

They started with a session exploring the unknown terrain of his body. His sensitive spots had definitely shifted. He was surprised to find that he was very aroused by being touched in some places far from the genital area. He kept looking for the erection, and Josephine kept telling him not to worry about it, but just to enjoy the touching. Their third touch session was spontaneous and involved touching of both partners.

Josephine also gave him more hugs and other spontaneous demonstrations of affection. She tried to wear clothes that appealed to him. Slowly, she "warmed him up" to the idea of lovemaking in a new way. She made sure she understood what made her feel good and guided him to the appropriate places, told him how to touch her for the greatest pleasure. They tried things they had never done before: oral sex, manual stimulation, vibrators, lubricants, and other things they didn't want to tell us in detail. And they always kept touching.

When Viagra came out, Napoleon tried it, but he got bad headaches. His doctor recommended shots, and Napoleon now takes tri-mix about once a month. The rest of the time he and Josephine engage in their newfound variety of lovemaking. They dress up a little for each other and make occasional "dates" with each other.

Napoleon comments, "It's almost embarrassing to think that we're in our sixties trying all these new things, but it has really recharged our batteries. In some ways we're like newlyweds now. I never knew I had such a sexy wife." Josephine says, "I have really great orgasms, and I'm not shy about showing him. It's important that he knows how much pleasure he gives me." But what's most important to her is that she was able to break through the barrier that had been created by Napoleon's pain over the erectile dysfunction.

The examples of these couples show that if you're interested in rebuilding your physical relationship, you can do it. The key ingredients are an understanding of your partner, the understanding of each other's bodies and likes and dislikes, creativity, and the willingness to try new things. A lot of touching and slowing down the pace of your lovemaking also help most couples. Love and caring for each other, and a sense of romance and adventure can revive the sizzle in your relationship. Treat each other as the sexual beings you are, and enjoy it!

We wish that each one of you will achieve the potential that you have. Cervantes wrote, "If only dreams and reality weren't so far apart." We submit that when you want good loving, you can realize your dream.

We wish you a happy, healthy, romantic, and loving relationship!

—Barbara and Ralph Alterowitz

APPENDICES

Appendix A
Manufacturers of
Erectile Dysfunction
Products

American MedTech
Penile splints
Brand name: Rejoyn
Vacuum pumps
Brand name: Rejoyn
  2124 University Avenue
  St. Paul, MN 55114
  Tel: 888-209-8609
      651-659-2406
  Web: www.rejoyn.com

Encore Medical Products Inc.
Vacuum pump
Brand name: Encore
  1002 North Central Expressway
  Suite 341
  Richardson, TX 75080
  Tel: 800-221-6603
  email: encoreved@aol.com

Harvard Scientific
Liposomal applied product
  1325 Airmotive Way, Suite 125
  Reno, NV 89502
  Tel: 775-323-6751
  Web: www.harvardscientific.com

ICOS
Oral medication
  22021 20th Avenue S.E.
  Bothell, WA 98021
  Tel: 206-485-1900
  Web: www.icos.com

MacroChem
Topical applied product
Brand name: Topiglan
  110 Hartwell Avenue, Suite 2
  Lexington, MA 02421-3134
  Tel: 781-862-4003
  Web: www.mchm.com
  www.macrochem.com

Mentor Urology, Inc.
Vacuum pumps
(Product line acquired by Vetco)
  5425 Hollister Avenue
  Santa Barbara, CA 93111
  Tel: 800-328-3863
      800-525-8161

Mission Pharmacal
Vacuum pumps
Brand name: VED
  10999 IH-10 West, Suite 1000
  San Antonio, TX 78230-1355
      or
  PO Box 786099
  San Antonio, TX 78278-6099
  Tel: 800-292-7364
  Web: www.missionpharmacal.com

NexMed
Topical cream
Brand name: Alprox-TD
   350 Corporate Blvd.
   Robinsville, NJ 08691
   Tel: 609-208-9688
   Web: www.nexmedinc.com

Pfizer Inc.
Oral medication
Brand name: Viagra
   235 East 42nd Street
   New York, NY 10007-5755
   Tel: 888-4-VIAGRA
   Web: www.viagra.com

Pharmacia-Upjohn
Injection medication
Brand name: Caverject
   95 Corporate Ave.
   Bridgewater, NJ   08807
   Tel: 800-253-8600
   Web: www.impotent.com

Pos-T-Vac
Vacuum pump
Brand Name: IVP
   1701 North 14th Avenue
   P.O. Box 1436
   Dodge City, KS 67801
   Tel: 800-279-7434
   Web: www.postvac.com

Schering-Plough
Oral medication
See Zonagen (Vasomax)
Licensed from Zonagen

Schwarz Pharma
Injection medication
Brand Name: EDEX
  6140 W. Executive Drive
  Mequon, WI 53092
  Tel: 800-558-5114
  Web: www.schwarzusa.com

Senetek
Injection medication
Brand name: Invicorp
  620 Airpark Road
  Napa, CA 94558
  Tel: 707-226-3900
  Web: www.senetekplc.com

TAP Pharmaceuticals
Oral medication
Brand name: UPRIMA
  2355 Waukegan Road
  Deerfield, IL 60015
  Tel: 800-348-2779
  Web: www.tapurology.com

Timm Medical
Vacuum pumps
Brand name: Osbon
  6585 City West Parkway
  Eden Prairie, MN 55344
  Tel: 800-438-8592
  Web: www.erectionsolutions.com

Vetco Inc.
Vacuum pumps
Brand name: Vetco and Mentor
  3700th Avenue S.
  Birmingham, AL 35222
  Tel: 800-827-8382
  Web: www.vetcoinc.com

VIVUS Inc.
Intraurethral suppository
Brand name: MUSE
    605 E. Fairchild Drive
    Mountain View, CA 94043
    Tel: 888-367-6873
    Web: www.vivus.com

Zonagen
Oral medication
Brand name: Vasomax
    2408 Timberlock Place
    Suite B-4
    Licensed to Schering-Plough
    The Woodlands, TX 77380
    Tel: 281-367-5892
    Web: www.zonagen.com

Appendix B
Resources for
Erectile Dysfunction

American Association of Sex Educators, Counselors,
and Therapists (AASECT)
P.O. Box 238
Mount Vernon, IA 52314-0238
Enclose self-addressed business-size envelope for list.

American Counseling Association (ACA)
American Association for Marriage and Family Therapy
1717 K Street, Suite 407
Washington, DC 20006
202-452-0109

Impotence Institute International
87-119 South Ruth Street
Maryville, TN 37801-5764

Impotence World Organization
Impotence Institute of America (IIA)
PO Box 410
Bowie, MD 20718-0410
800-669-1603; 301-262-2400

Sexual Function Health Council
American Foundation for Urologic Disease
1128 North Charles Street
Baltimore, MD 21201
800-232-7688

Sexuality Information and Education Council of the
United States (SIECUS)
130 West 42nd Street
Suite 350
New York, NY 10036
212-819-9770

The National Women's Health Resource Center
120 Albany Street
Suite 820
New Brunswick, NJ 08901
877-986-9742

The Geddings Osbon Foundation
P.O. Box 1593
Augusta, GA 30903
800-433-4215

Further Reading

Books

Eid, J. François, *Making Love Again: Regaining Sexual Potency*, Brunner-Mazel, New York, 1993.

Hellstrom, Wayne J.G., M.D., Editor, *The Handbook of Sexual Dysfunction*, The American Society of Andrology, San Francisco, CA 1999

Jacobowitz, Ruth S., *150 Most-Asked Questions about Midlife Sex, Love and Intimacy*, Hearst, New York, 1995.

Levinson, Daniel J., *The Seasons of a Man's Life*, Ballantine Books, New York, 1979.

Love, Patricia, PH.D., and Jo Robinson, *Hot Monogamy*, Plume-Penguin, New York, 1994.

Masters, William H., and Virginia E. Johnson, *The Pleasure Bond*, Little, Brown, Boston, 1974.

Ornish, Dean, *Love and Survival*, HarperCollins, New York, 1998.

Padma-Nathan, Harin, M.D., *Medical Management of Erectile Dysfunction: A Primary-Care Manual*, Professional Communications, Inc., 1999

Pilgrim, Aubrey, *A Revolutionary Approach to Prostate Cancer*, Sterling House, Pittsburgh, PA, 1998.

Reid, Daniel P., *The Tao of Health, Sex, and Longevity*, Simon & Schuster, New York, 1989.

Ryan, George, *Reclaiming Male Sexuality*. M. Evans, New York, 1997.

Schnarch, David, Ph.D., *Passions in Marriage*. Henry Holt, New York, 1997.

Vaughan, Susan C., M.D., *Viagra: A Guide to the Phenomenal Potency-Promoting Drug,* Pocket Books, New York, 1998.

Waldman, Mark Robert, *The Art of Staying Together,* Tarcher-Putnam, New York, 1998.

Wallerstein, Judith S., *The Good Marriage: How and Why Love Lasts,* Warner Books, 1996.

Scientific and Technical Papers

Broderick, Gregory A., Craig F. Donatucci, et al., *Male Sexual Dysfunction: Diagnostic and Treatment Options,* American Urological Association, 93rd Annual Meeting, June 1998, 80 pp.

Burnett, Arthur L., *Erectile Dysfunction: A Practical Approach for Primary Care,* Geriatrics, Vol. 53, No. 2, February 1998.

Burnett, Arthur L., Neurophysiology of Erectile Function and Dysfunction, *The Handbook of Sexual Dysfunction,* American Society of Andrology, 1999.

Donatucci, C. F., Prosexual Drugs: Oral and Topical Agents for Enhancing Erectile and Ejaculatory Control, *Male Sexual Dysfunction: Diagnostic and Treatment Options,* American Urological Association, 1998 Annual Meeting.

Geary, E. Stewart, Theresa E. Dendinger, et al., Nerve Sparing Radical Prostatectomy: A Different View, *Journal of Urology,* July 1995, Vol. 154, pp. 145-149

Hanash, Kamal A., Comparative Results of Goal Oriented Therapy for Erectile Dysfunction, *Journal of Urology,* June 1997, Vol. 157, pp. 2135-38.

Helgason, A. R., et al., Distress Due to Unwanted Side Effects of Prostate Cancer Treatment Is Related to Impaired Well-Being (Quality of Life), *Prostate Cancer and Prostatic Diseases,* June 1998, Vol. 1, No. 3, p. 128.

Helgason, Asgeir R., et al., Factors Associated With Waning Sexual Function Among Elderly Men And Prostate Cancer Patients, Journal of Urology, Vol. 158, pp. 155-59, July 1997.

National Institutes of Health, Impotence, *NIH Consensus Statement Online*, National Institutes of Health, December 7-9, 1992, 10(4): 1-31.

Jarow , Jonathan P., Patrick Nana-Sinkam, et al., Outcome Analysis of Goal Directed Therapy For Impotence, *Journal of Urology*, May 1996, pp. 1609-12.

Kim, Edward D., and Larry I. Lipshultz, Advances in the Treatment of Organic Erectile Dysfunction, *Hospital Practice*, April 15, 1997, pp. 101-20.

Kirby, R. S., Medical Management of BPH: Where are we going?, *Prostate Cancer and Prostatic Diseases*, March 1999, Vol. 2, No. 2, pp. 62-65

Kirby, R. S., et al., Prostate Cancer and Sexual Function, *Prostate Cancer and Prostatic Diseases,* June 1998, Vol. 1, No. 4, p. 183

Laumann, Edward O., Anthony Paik, et al., Sexual Dysfunction in the United States: Prevalence and Predictors, *Journal of the American Medical Association*, Vol. 281, No. 6, pp. 537-44

Litwin, M. S., and D. F. Penson, Health-Related Quality of Life in Men with Prostate Cancer, *Prostate Cancer and Prostatic Diseases,* June 1998, Vol. 1, No. 5, p. 228.

Morales, Alvaro, Jeremy P. W. Heaton, et al., Oral and Topical Treatment of Erectile Dysfunction: Present and Future, *Urologic Clinics of North America,* Vol. 22, No. 4, November 1995, pp. 879-86.

Melman, Arnold, Impotence in the Age of Viagra, *Scientific American Presents*, Summer 1999, pp. 62-67.

Myers, Robert P., Editorial: Prostate Cancer — Neurovascular Preservation; Smoking Cessation May Enhance Prognosis?, *The Journal of Urology*, Vol. 154, July 1995, pp. 158-59.

Nehra, Ajay, Oxygen Levels and Their Effect on Erectile Function, *Family Urology,* Winter 1997, p. 19.

Quinlan, David M., Jonathan I. Epstein, et al., Sexual Function Following Radical Prostatectomy: Influence of Preservation of Neurovascular Bundles, *Journal Of Urology,* Vol. 145, 998-1002.

Penson, D. F., Transitions in Health-Related Quality of Life during the First Nine Months after Diagnosis with Prostate Cancer, *Prostate Cancer and Prostatic Diseases,* June 1998, Vol. 1, No. 3, p. 134.

Rosen, Raymond, Ph.D., Irwin Goldstein, et al., *A Process of Care Model,* The University of Medicine and Dentistry (UMDNJ) — Robert Wood Johnson Medical School, 1998.

Schover, Leslie R., Ph.D., Sexual Rehabilitation after Treatment for Prostate Cancer, *Cancer Supplement,* February 1, 1993, Vol. 71, No. 3, pp. 1024-30.

Zonszein, Joel, Diagnosis and Management of Endocrine Disorders of Erectile Dysfunction, *Urologic Clinics of North America,* Vol. 22, No. 4, November 1995, pp. 789-802

Feedback

Dear Reader:

We hope *The Lovin' Ain't Over* has been helpful to you. We value your comments and would appreciate your taking a few minutes to share your thoughts with us so that we can help future readers.

Please send your feedback to:
Ralph and Barbara Alterowitz
P.O. Box 1388
Bethesda, MD 20827-1388
e-mail:edbook@ibm.net

1. What parts of this book did you find most useful?

_____

_____

2. What parts of this book did you find least useful?

_____

_____

3. In your own situation, what techniques and approaches have you found to be most useful?

_____

_____

least useful?

_____

_____

4. Are there any topics, concerns, or issues we overlooked?

_____

_____

5. Do you have any suggestions that we should pass on to:

Survivors and partners?

_____

_____

Physicians?

_____

_____

Counselors?

_____

_____

Researchers?

_____

_____

6. Please use this section or a separate sheet of paper for any other comments you wish to make on the contents of this book.

If you are interested in receiving more information on this subject as it becomes available, please give us your name and address. Your information will not be provided to others.

Name_____

Address_____

Telephone_____

email_____

Preferred means of contact: mail____ email____

telephone ____

Feedback

Dear Reader:

We hope *The Lovin' Ain't Over* has been helpful to you. We value your comments and would appreciate your taking a few minutes to share your thoughts with us so that we can help future readers.

Please send your feedback to:

Ralph and Barbara Alterowitz
P.O. Box 1388
Bethesda, MD 20827-4006
e-mail:edbook@ibm.net

1. What parts of this book did you find most useful?

_____

_____

2. What parts of this book did you find least useful?

_____

_____

3. In your own situation, what techniques and approaches have you found to be most useful?

_____

_____

least useful?

_____

_____

4. Are there any topics, concerns, or issues we overlooked?

_____

_____

5. Do you have any suggestions that we should pass on to:

Survivors and partners?

_____

_____

Physicians?

_____

_____

Counselors?

_____

_____

Researchers?

_____

_____

6. Please use this section or a separate sheet of paper for any other comments you wish to make on the contents of this book.

If you are interested in receiving more information on this subject as it becomes available, please give us your name and address. Your information will not be provided to others.

Name_____

Address_____

Telephone_____

email_____

Preferred means of contact: mail_____ email_____

telephone _____

About the Authors

Separately and together, Barbara and Ralph Alterowitz have worked with support groups and counseled prostate cancer patients and survivors and their partners on coping with the diagnosis, treatment, and aftereffects of prostate cancer. Finding that there was a big information gap when dealing with impotence, Barbara and Ralph overcame their natural reluctance to discuss sexuality in public. Since 1997, they have teamed up to educate couples on how to reestablish intimacy, loving, and communication when faced with the effects of prostate disease and treatment. During this period, they have talked to hundreds of individuals and couples about sexuality and prostate disease.

Ralph is a prostate cancer survivor and activist. He was the founding vice-chair and a former director of the National Prostate Cancer Coalition (NPCC) and a founder and president of the Education Center for Prostate Cancer Patients (ECPCP).

Ralph brings to this topic a background that includes more than 20 years of medical experience, e.g. the delivery of health care in the field, the design and implementation of high-tech medical systems, and health care studies. Currently, he is president of Venture Tech Corporation, an international consulting practice specializing in business start-ups and the creation of technology partnerships, with a focus on the health care industry. He is also an author, educator, and speaker on the subject of entrepreneurship and venturing.

Barbara's professional background includes sales and marketing of technology products and services, research into new business start-up models and corporate leveraging through business alliances. In her "day job," Barbara is a marketing executive with a major high-tech company.

Barbara and Ralph have been happily married for 16 years.

Index